Darwin In Ilkley

Darwin In Ilkley

Mike Dixon & Gregory Radick

For Mark, Jane and Anna Dixon
and
Ben and Matthew Radick

First published 2009
Reprinted 2014

The History Press
The Mill, Brimscombe Port
Stroud, Gloucestershire, GL5 2QG
www.thehistorypress.co.uk

ISBN 978 0 7524 5283 8

Typesetting and origination by The History Press
Printed and bound in Great Britain by
Marston Book Services Limited, Oxfordshire

Contents

About the Authors

Mike Dixon is Emeritus Professor of Gastrointestinal Pathology at the University of Leeds and has lived in Ilkley since 1970. In parallel with a distinguished clinical and academic career in Pathology, he pursued a keen interest in local history. The introduction of hydropathy and the Victorian development of Ilkley are particular interests, and through them he came to study the town's most illustrious water cure patient, Charles Darwin. This involvement in local history has led to the publication of *Images of England: Ilkley* (1999) and *Ilkley – History and Guide* (2002).

Gregory Radick is Senior Lecturer in History and Philosophy of Science at the University of Leeds and has lived in Ilkley since 2000. His interests as a historian have centred on Darwin's theory of evolution, its historical contexts and its legacies within and beyond biology. Previous books include *The Simian Tongue: The Long Debate About Animal Language* (2007) and, as co-editor (with Jonathan Hodge), *The Cambridge Companion to Darwin* (second edition, 2009). Currently he is researching the early years of Mendelian genetics.

Preface

On 4 October 1859, Charles Darwin arrived in Ilkley to take the 'water cure'. At that time, Ilkley was no more than a village, similar to many others in the old West Riding of Yorkshire but distinguished from them by its hydropathic establishments. Darwin stayed for just nine weeks; but it was during this visit that his famous book *On the Origin of Species by Means of Natural Selection* was published. A man who was already recognised as a gifted naturalist and scientific voyager was on the verge of becoming one of the most influential, celebrated and controversial figures of all time. The publication of the *Origin* on 24 November 1859 marked the start of Darwin's new identity as a theorist of evolution.

Darwin's visit to Ilkley attracts only brief mention in recent biographies.[1] Yet the visit coincided with an important period in Darwin's life. During his time in Ilkley, he had to cope with chronic illness and the rigours of the water cure, make the final corrections to the text of the *Origin*, and manage the reception of a book that he had come to refer to as his 'abominable volume'.[2] We shall examine the scenes of all this intense activity: Wells House Hydropathic Establishment, including the treatments, amenities and Darwin's fellow guests; the social life of the Hydro and his participation in it; the austere surroundings of North House, a temporary residence made bearable by the presence of his family; and Ilkley itself, rustic and inaccessible, but a Northern Mecca for the 'water patient'.

That Darwin came to Ilkley to undergo the water cure raises intriguing questions. How was it that a man of his scientific calibre was drawn to a treatment that many at the time considered to be quackery? Why did he feel compelled to travel over two hundred miles from Down House in Kent to a village in Yorkshire to undergo this treatment, which was available much closer to home? In answering these questions, we will also consider the mysterious nature of Darwin's illness and the well-documented failure of orthodox treatments. Darwin's experiences of the water cure regime in Ilkley turn out to disclose evidence that, we suggest, may allow a final settling of the debate over what ailed him.

Attention to Darwin's life in Ilkley likewise throws new light on the intellectual run-up to the *Origin*'s publication. The unparalleled examination offered in these pages of Darwin's Ilkley correspondence reveals a mixture of trepidation at the book's likely reception and assertiveness over the correctness of his theory. Against the backdrop of the moor, Darwin took part in one of the most challenging debates that he would ever enter into over the *Origin*, touching on everything from whether he had relegated God to an implausibly small role in the making of new species to whether domesticated dogs have more than one wild ancestor (a politically charged question at that moment).

Taken together, these reconstructions give us a composite portrait of a man who, far from the cringing recluse of legend, comes across here as warm, convivial and socially and intellectually confident. Yet for all that Darwin is at the centre, the book is also a work of local history. From 1859 onwards numerous hydropathic hotels were opened in Ilkley, leading to an upsurge in visitors and providing additional employment. The hotels also encouraged an expansion of shops and services in the town, and the population grew – albeit slowly at first. Rapid growth followed the opening of the railway lines to Leeds and Bradford in 1865. Thus at the time of Darwin's visit, Ilkley was in its last years as a minor spa. Over the next decade, its new transport links and a marked increase in house building would change it into a commuter town, as well as a fashionable inland resort.

We feel, therefore, that it is both fitting and timely to give a detailed account of Darwin's short but eventful visit to a small Yorkshire village that was itself on the cusp of 'transmutation'.

Notes

1   In Bowlby, J., *Charles Darwin: A New Life* (W.W. Norton & Co., New York 1991) less than two of 466 pages of text are devoted to the Ilkley visit, and in Desmond, A., and Moore, J., *Darwin* (Michael Joseph, London 1991) there are just over two of 677 text pages on the subject. In her biography, Janet Browne gives a more detailed account but this only extends to eight of 497 text pages in the second volume of her two-volume work, (Browne, J., *Charles Darwin: The Power of Place*, Jonathan Cape, London 2002).

2   'So much for my abominable volume, which has cost me so much labour that I almost hate it', C.D. to W.D. Fox, 23 Sept 1859; Correspondence (see Abbreviations, p. 10).

In the published Correspondence the date of the letter is given in a standard form, but those elements not taken directly from the letter text are supplied in square brackets.

Acknowledgements

The authors thank:

Dr Roger Pyrah of Skipton, who in May 1988 first alerted Mike Dixon to Charles Darwin's visit to Ilkley, and for his continuing interest in Darwin's illness.

Alex Cockshott for information regarding Wells House and Wells Terrace, and the photograph of Marshall Hainsworth. Dennis Warwick and Brian Clayton for genealogical information concerning the Hainsworth family, and Jean Hawley and Anne Sanders for information concerning South View and Laburnum Cottage.

Colin Clarkson for access to the title deeds of Rombald's Hotel and maps relating to its period as Usher's boarding house.

Peter J. Adams of Heritage Cartography for permission to publish the map of Ilkley in 1859, modified from his 1847 version.

Petr Neugebauer, Priessnitzovy Lécebné Lázne Ltd, for permission to reproduce illustrations relating to the practice of Vinzenz Priessnitz in Jesenik.

The late Kate Mason for details relating to White Wells in the Addingham records, and the late Chris Hellier of the Museum of Farnham for information relating to Moor Park, Surrey.

Thanks are due to the staff of Ilkley Public Library, to Kathryn Emmott, Sandra Hanby and the late Roland Wade for photographs, and to May Pickles for the etching of Ben Rhydding Hydro. We are particularly indebted to the late Gordon Burton and his wife Betty, for the loan of items from his unique collection of old Ilkley photographs. All unattributed photographs are from Mike Dixon's collection.

Finally we wish to thank Gerry Shaper for spurring us to action in time for the anniversary of Darwin's visit to Ilkley, and Lindsay Gledhill, Jon Hodge and Jo Lawton for their perceptive and helpful comments on the manuscript.

Abbreviations:

We have used the following abbreviations in the sources and notes at the end of each chapter:

C.D. – Charles Darwin

Autobiography – Nora Barlow, Ed. *The autobiography of Charles Darwin, 1809-1882, with original omissions restored.* (Collins, London: 1958).

Correspondence – Frederick H. Burkhardt, Sydney Smith, et al., Eds. *The Correspondence of Charles Darwin, vols 1 – 14* (Cambridge University Press, Cambridge: 1983-2004).

DCP – Darwin Correspondence Project; www.darwinproject.ac.uk. This source is used for recently discovered letters that do not appear in the published Correspondence. Each letter in the catalogue has a unique identifying number.

Life and Letters – Francis Darwin, Ed. *The Life and Letters of Charles Darwin. Vols. I-III* (John Murray, London: 1887).

Journal – Darwin's personal 'Journal' (Cambridge University Library DAR 158) is available online (www.darwin-online.org.uk) but has also been transcribed and reproduced as appendices ('Chronology') in the published volumes of Correspondence.

Chapter One

First Impressions

I am in the establishment & have a sitting room and bedroom. I always hate everything new & perhaps it is only this that makes me at present detest the whole place & everybody except one kind lady here, whom I knew at Moor Park. – It would be excessively nice if you were to come here for a time. Dr Smith, I think, is sensible, but he is a Homoeopathist!! & as far as I can judge does not personally look much after patients or anything else. – There is a capital steward & the House seems well managed.[1]

So wrote Charles Darwin from Wells House Hydropathic Hotel on Thursday 6 October, two days after his arrival in Ilkley. His correspondent, the clergyman and naturalist William Fox, was a close friend from his Cambridge days (indeed a second cousin), now living in Cheshire – at that time, about five hours journey from Ilkley. These opening lines in Darwin's first surviving letter from Ilkley touch on two key elements of his visit: the hotel itself, and the people he encountered there.

Built three years before Darwin's visit, Wells House still stands, having recently been converted into apartments. The building occupies a prominent position 300ft above the centre of Ilkley. When the hotel was built, Ilkley was little more than a small collection of streets and houses straddling the main Otley to Skipton turnpike on the south side of the River Wharfe. Wells House was not the first hydropathic hotel to be built in the Ilkley area. That distinction goes to Ben Rhydding Hydropathic Hotel, opened in 1844, an even larger edifice a mile down the valley. By the late 1840s, Ben Rhydding was seen to be manifestly successful. The owner, Dr William MacLeod, was a charismatic figure who had established a considerable reputation for his 'water cure', and large numbers of patients visited the establishment – the first purpose-built hydropathic hotel in England.[2]

Others sought to follow his example, but the lack of availability of suitable building sites put a bar on such developments. Apart from smallholdings in the centre of the town, much of the land in Ilkley was in the ownership of the hereditary Lords of the Manor, the Middeltons. Successive Lords of the Manor had resolutely opposed any sale of land, but by 1850 the family were facing serious financial difficulties and they became more receptive to such proposals. In October that year, the then Lord of the Manor, Peter Middelton, was approached by the representative of a group of 'commercial gentlemen' with an offer to purchase nine acres

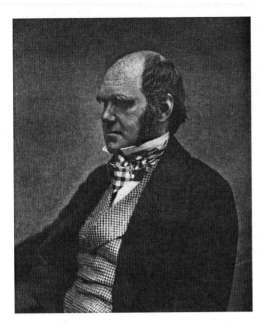

Charles Darwin: a portrait taken by Messrs Maull and Polyblank. The date of the photograph is uncertain, but it has been claimed that it was taken when Darwin was aged fifty, dating it to 1859 – the year that he visited Ilkley. (Hulton Archive – Getty Images)

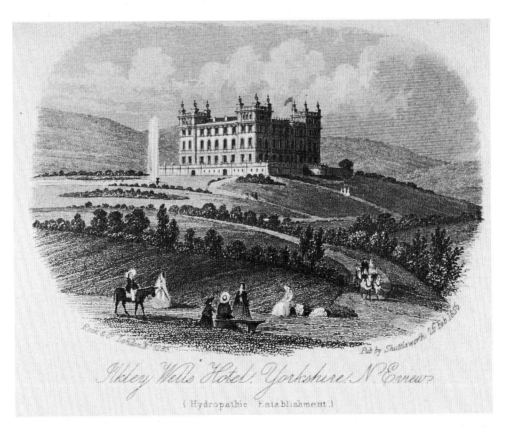

Wells House Hotel, February 1856. An idealised view of the hotel, which was not officially opened until May 1856, showing the possible layout of the gardens and drives, then under construction.

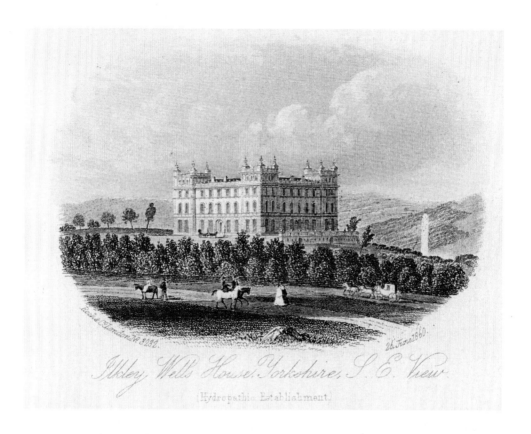

Ilkley Wells House, Yorkshire, S.E. View.
(Hydropathic Establishment.)

Above: Wells House in June 1860 with a more accurate representation of the approach and main entrance to the hotel. The east terrace, which contained the treatment rooms beneath it (accessed at basement level from the hotel), is clearly shown.

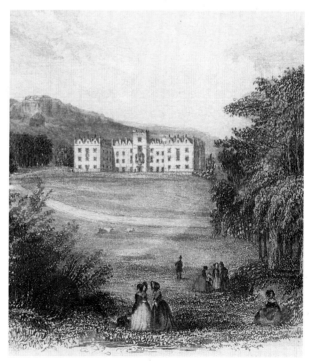

Right: Ben Rhydding Hydro, Ilkley's first hydropathic hotel, was built high above the then hamlet of Wheatley beneath the Cow and Calf Rocks. (May Pickles)

of land at the top of Wells Road.[3] The land comprised two large fields – Little and Great Intake[4] – surrounding a dilapidated former cotton-mill (by then converted into three shabby cottages rented by the Hodgson family).[5] Since the annual rent from the land and cottages only amounted to £14, the offer of £4,000 by the joint-stock company was a bargain too good to miss. Thomas Constable, the Otley solicitor acting for the Middeltons, urged acceptance of the offer, 'not only because £4,000 is an enormous price for nine acres of inferior hillside land, but still more because the establishment will be tenanted by wealthy and numerous occupiers whose wants will greatly enhance the value of all the adjoining property'. Peter Middelton was persuaded but, partly as a consequence of conveyancing difficulties, the transaction was not finalised until 8 June 1854.[6] In order to secure a plentiful supply of pure water for their hydropathic hotel, the developers also purchased a direct supply from the spring behind the old bath-house, White Wells, on the hillside above the site of the proposed hotel. Spring water was diverted via an underground cistern near the bath-house and then led underground through a 1in diameter pipe down to the hotel.[7]

The developers had their land and a water supply, now they set about appointing an architect. In a bold and inspired choice, they settled on a young Leeds architect, Cuthbert Brodrick, who already had one magnificent design in his growing portfolio – Leeds Town Hall. Indeed, building of the Town Hall was in progress when he undertook to design the hotel in Ilkley. Brodrick was brought up in Hull, and at the age of sixteen (in 1837) was apprenticed there to a highly successful practice belonging to Henry Francis Lockwood. In 1845 he set up his own practice in Hull

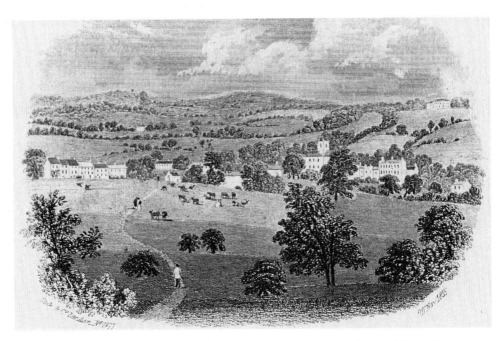

Ilkley from the Cow Pastures, 1855. This artist's impression shows a rustic village with little of note apart from the tower of the parish church and the large house on the opposite hill side – Myddelton Lodge, home of the Lord of the Manor. The houses on the left mark the line of Wells Road leading up to the moor and to Wells House.

and was responsible for several local projects, including the splendid Royal Institution building completed in 1854. Two years earlier, he had won an open competition for the design of Leeds Town Hall – with a prize of £200 – and had moved his office to Park Row in Leeds.[8] Despite his comparative youthfulness, Brodrick was a highly sophisticated architect. During his years in Hull, he took several months leave of absence to undertake a 'Grand Tour' of the European capitals. This exposure to continental influences was to inform his designs in ways that were beyond the experience of his provincial competitors.[9] His design for Wells House embodied much of his flair for restrained grandeur. The style revealed Brodrick's Italian influences, being reminiscent of a palazzo in the form of a square with towers at each corner and a central courtyard. Unfortunately, his restraint in design did not extend to the cost. The completed project cost in the region of £30,000, equivalent to at least £3 million pounds in today's values.

By February 1856, the directors were sufficiently confident about their scheme to issue a 'news story' via the *Leeds Mercury*:[10]

Ilkley Wells:– To many of our readers these words bring to mind an irregular whitewashed building, about half way up the hills above Ilkley, containing two formidable looking wells, or plunge baths, into which the strong minded searchers after health have been in the habit of immersing themselves and their families these hundred years and more. But time works wonders – for now, when he hears of "Ilkley Wells," instead of associating this humble though venerable pile, the reader must picture to himself a stately edifice, a veritable Italian palace, which now claims that name, and which,

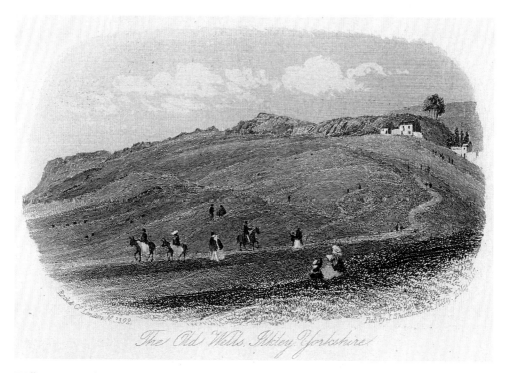

The Old Wells, Ilkley, Yorkshire

Wells House was built close to the foot of the donkey track leading up to the old bath-house on the moor, White Wells. Guests with a south-facing bedroom would have enjoyed a view similar to this.

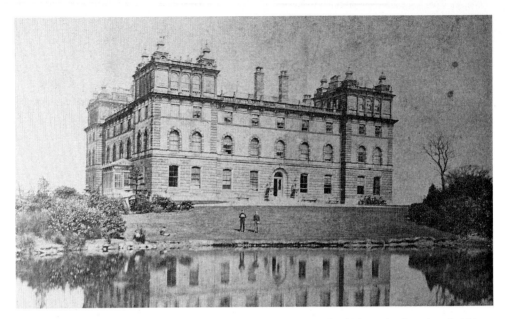

Wells House Hydro in the 1860s. The hotel, seen from across the artificial lake at the front (south side), would have appeared like this at the time of Darwin's visit. (Ilkley Public Library)

during two years past, has been gradually rearing its towers above the lovely valley of the Wharfe. Health and relaxation, cold water and creature comforts, appear to have been the object in view with the projectors of this bold undertaking.

The building is designed for a hydropathic establishment and hotel, and, truly, the votaries of hydropathy and the frequenters of watering-place hotels may search far and wide before they find a resting-place to compare in architectural effect with this noble structure. It stands not very far distant from the Old Wells, which still remain to assert their ancient title, and which share with it the waters of their crystal spring. The situation is thus very happily chosen, as all frequenters of Ilkley will know, who remember the charming views from this position on the hill. If pure cold water and free bracing air can do much towards restoring health, certainly the new Hydropathic Establishment will be in possession of two important remedies; and summer tourists will have another object added to the list of attractions in hill and valley scenery… At present the place presents a busy scene of preparation, both in the house and grounds, but it is said that all will be complete in readiness for the approaching season.

The building was completed by May 1856. The elevated site (Wells House is 517ft above sea-level) had two main advantages; firstly, the 'bracing air' at this height was claimed as an important adjunct to the water cure regime, and secondly, the building formed a striking feature of the landscape and could be seen from almost everywhere in the vicinity. The main entrance was on the south side facing the moor, and a curved drive led down to the extended Wells Road, a road linking it directly to the centre of the town. The house was surrounded by gardens laid out by the celebrated landscape gardener Joshua Major, who had been responsible for the design of Manchester's first three municipal parks.[11] In addition to decorative flower

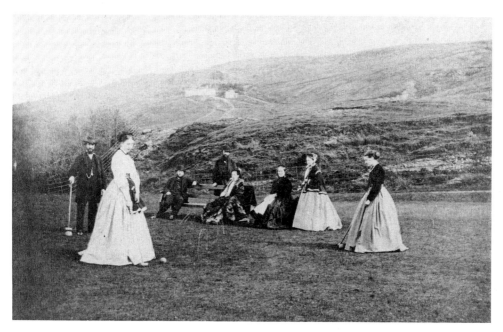

Guests enjoy a game of croquet at Wells House in the 1860s. (Ilkley Public Library)

beds and paths, many trees and shrubs were planted, and lawns laid out for tennis and croquet. Two small lakes opposite the entrance of the hotel completed the scene.

The hotel had its own stables, which were built on the site of the old cotton mill. The stalls for the horses and storage accommodation for the carriages were arranged around a large central yard whose entrance was flanked by two cottages, a porter's lodge and a house for the gardener.

Internally, no expense had been spared in the furnishing and equipping of the bedrooms and public rooms. The hotel had 'a dining room capable of seating between 80 and 100 guests, a large public drawing room, a private drawing room for ladies only, and a coffee room for general visitors or those not wanting to join the company at the table d'hote, a billiard room, thirteen private sitting rooms, eighty-seven bedrooms and six bathrooms'.[12] Although viewed from our perspective the number of bathrooms seems grossly inadequate, the Victorian hotel relied on bedrooms having movable, rather than plumbed-in fittings. The usual practice was to wash or bathe in one's own room, and on request a chambermaid would bring hot water to fill a bowl on the wash-stand or provide a hip-bath. Likewise, a midnight hike to some distant lavatory was circumvented by use of the bedside commode.

The hotel corridors were spacious and well-lit. Walking around the corridors formed a valuable alternative to outdoor exercise when the weather was poor – an essential facility in Ilkley. The treatment rooms occupied the extensive basement under the terrace on the east of the building. They contained a variety of baths, douches, massage and wet-sheet tables. The marble walls and the richly patterned tiles provided a suitably opulent backcloth for the watery arts of the hydropathic practitioner.

The building was officially opened on 28 May 1856 when 'about 150 ladies and gentlemen partook of a sumptuous collation, most tastefully served in the large dining hall, under the

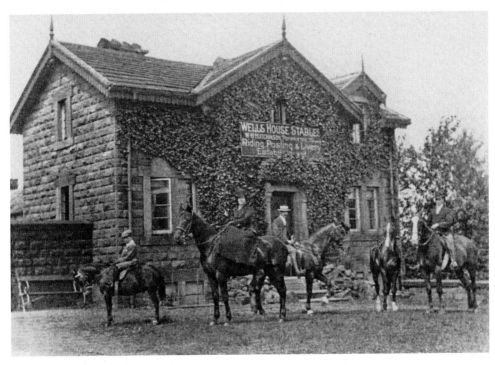

Wells House Stables. One of the two cottages that flanked the entrance to the stable yard, photographed in the 1890s. The cottage, 'Ivy Lodge', has been enlarged recently and is now a private house.

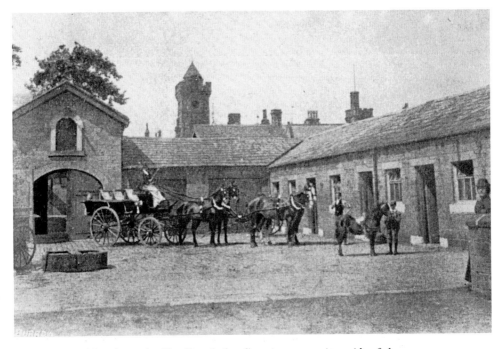

Wells House Stables. The yard, with a 'four-in-hand' carriage occupying pride of place.

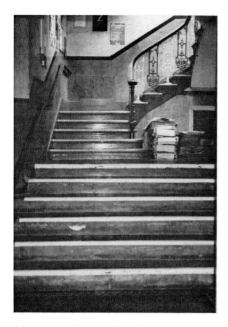

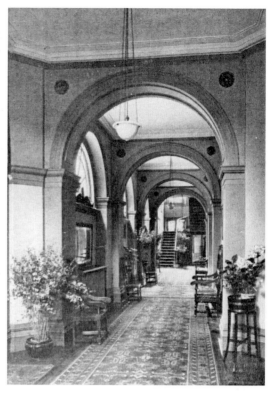

The staircase leading from the ground floor of the hotel down to the baths and treatment rooms situated below the east terrace. Photograph taken in 1999, prior to the redevelopment of the building and conversion into apartments. (Kathryn Emmott)

Ground floor corridor in Wells House photographed in the 1930s.

direction of the manager, Mr Strachan. To enliven the proceedings the band of the North York Rifles played during the splendid repast'.[12] The host at this celebratory meal was the chairman of the board of directors, a redoubtable Bradford wine and spirit merchant, Benjamin Briggs Popplewell.[13] The 'top table', which must have been a long one, was made up of fellow directors and their wives, civic dignitaries, clergymen and people otherwise connected with the enterprise, like Cuthbert Brodrick and the Middelton's solicitor, Thomas Constable.[14]

Despite this ambitious start, all did not go well for Mr Popplewell and his fellow directors. Guests were not attracted in the numbers required and the enterprise was soon in financial difficulties. Some of the blame was levelled at the resident physician, Dr Antoine Rischanek, a 'water-doctor' from Vienna who had presided over a similarly unsuccessful period after the opening of Ben Rhydding Hydropathic Hotel. Two years after his appointment there, he had been dismissed and, after a year's inter-regnum, replaced by Dr Macleod, who had gone on to make such a success of the place.[14] Now, Rischanek was to suffer a similar fate. He departed in April 1858 and was immediately replaced by a doctor from Sheffield with an interest in hydropathy, Dr Edmund Smith. As at Ben Rhydding, Rischanek's replacement appears to have turned around the fortunes of the place. By the summer of 1859, the hotel, and its physician, had managed to acquire a good reputation.

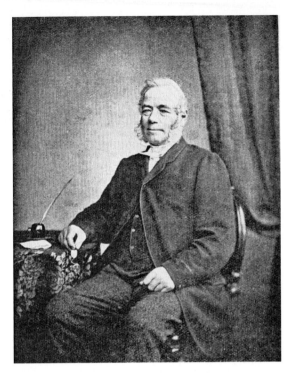

Benjamin Briggs Popplewell, Bradford
wine and spirits merchant and chairman
of the directors of the Wells House
Hydropathic Establishment.

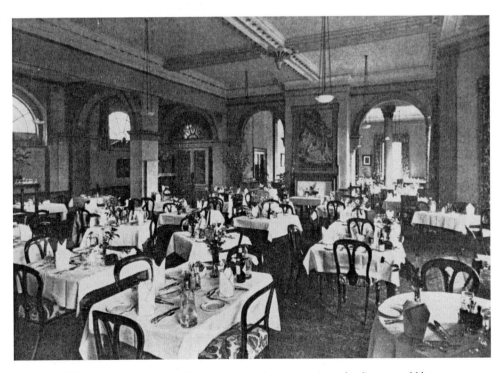

The main dining room photographed in the 1930s. In the Victorian era, the diners would have sat at
long, refectory-type tables.

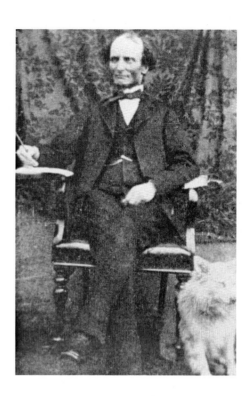

Dr Edmund Smith, physician at Wells House,
c. 1860. (Ilkley Public Library)

But Darwin was not much impressed by reputation, and the discovery that Dr Smith was a homoeopathist would have irritated him. He had a deep-seated antagonism towards homoeopathy – the administration of minute amounts of drugs in order to excite symptoms similar to those of the disease to be treated. Writing some years before to his Cheshire cousin Fox, Darwin made his views clear:

> You speak about Homoeopathy; which is a subject which makes me more wrath, even than does Clair-voyance: clairvoyance so transcends belief, that one's ordinary faculties are put out of the question, but in Homoeopathy common sense & common observation come into play, & both these must go to the Dogs, if the infinitesimal doses have any effect whatever.[15]

Edmund Smith practised for many years as an 'orthodox' medical practitioner before turning to homoeopathy. He had previously worked as a surgeon in the service of the Hudson Bay Company, and then acquired a medical practice in Sheffield.[16] The date of Dr Smith's 'conversion' to homoeopathy is not recorded but he is listed in the British Journal of Homoeopathy in 1850 and in the British and Foreign Homoeopathic Medical Directory and Record of 1855.[17] In 1858, he was created M.D. by the Archbishop of Canterbury – a so-called 'Lambeth degree', given in recognition of his medical experience but also an acknowledgement of his services to the Church of England. As regards his medical expertise, Dr Smith was not a shining example of the efficacy of either homoeopathy or the 'water cure', for he suffered chronic ill health and was debilitated throughout his time in Ilkley.[18] This could explain Darwin's observation that Dr Smith 'does not personally look much after patients or anything else'.[18]

Although the directors of Wells House had appointed Dr Smith as 'Medical Director and Manager', the latter title held an ambiguity.[19] Smith managed the patients but the hotel was managed by Henry Strachan, a man with over ten year's experience as House Steward at Ben Rhydding before joining the staff at Wells House.[20] Given that Darwin considered the place 'well managed', Strachan must have run a 'tight ship'. Wells House required the usual hotel personnel including a general housekeeper, a cook, kitchen maids, porters, waiters, chambermaids and gardeners, together with the male and female bath-attendants required for the hydropathic treatments.[21] The latter had to be carefully chosen. An air of decorum had to be maintained in the treatment rooms and, to this end, the attendants had to be mature and discreet. Female bath-attendants had to be 'respectable', 'not less than thirty years of age' and 'have had considerable experience'.[22]

Despite all this attention to detail, Darwin's initial reaction, as we have seen, was to 'detest the whole place'. Given the facilities at Wells House and the beauty of its setting, this must have been a highly unusual response. Darwin, however, was a highly unusual visitor. Over many years, he had become increasingly anxious when meeting new people, and by his own admission found social gatherings an ordeal. 'I find by dear bought experience that I cannot visit anywhere, as the excitement invariably does me harm for days afterwards'.[23] He wrote in 1852 of leading the life of a hermit,[24] and a year earlier had confessed that 'I very seldom leave home, as I find perfect quietude suits my health best'.[25] Darwin generally only left Down House (his home in Kent) reluctantly, and then in the company of his wife; he carefully controlled the number of visitors he saw, and normally shunned conversation with those outside his circle of family and close friends.[26]

Given this psychological background, it was no less than heroic for Darwin to make the solitary journey to Ilkley and to place himself in a large hydropathic establishment with its unappealing clientele, the sick and suffering of the upper-classes – the effete, the neurotic, the halt and the lame. Certainly the prospect filled him with foreboding. It was no doubt this dread of a house filled with strangers that prompted him to write to Miss Mary Butler, the 'kind lady' who had made an impression on him when he had stayed at Moor Park, a hydropathic establishment in Surrey, earlier that year.

Mary Butler was a charming Irish woman who regaled fellow guests at Moor Park with witty conversation and ghost stories.[27] She appears to have quickly won Charles Darwin's attention when he stayed there in February 1859. This is unsurprising; Darwin's weakness for attractive younger women was well known to his family. His son Francis Darwin recounted:

He was particularly charming when "chaffing" any one, and in high spirits over it. His manner at such times was light-hearted and boyish, and his refinement of nature came out most strongly. So, when he was talking to a lady who pleased and amused him, the combination of raillery and deference was delightful to see.[28]

A daughter, Henrietta Darwin, recalled that her father displayed a 'mixture of playfulness, deference, and admiration which made his manner so delightful to any woman who attracted him – with whom he was in love as he was pleased to call it. He was often in love with the heroines of the many novels that were read to him, and used always to maintain both in books and in real life that a touch of affectation was necessary to complete the charm of a pretty woman'.[29] Perhaps it was Mary Butler's affectation in placing a pile of salt on the table beside her plate, a practice shared by Darwin, which sparked some mutual attraction. Certainly following his stay at Moor Park he wrote her an affectionate and frivolous letter:

> I enjoyed my fortnight extremely at Moor Park, but if I were long exposed to the very pleasant temptation of sitting between Miss Craik & you, I wonder what I should not come to believe. Honeysuckles turning into oaks would be a mere trifle & new species turning up on every Railway embankment. [30]

The content and light-hearted tone of this single letter to Mary Butler is a revelation. Darwin, the self-confessed recluse of Down House, admits that his two weeks' stay at Moor Park had been extremely enjoyable. Indeed, he acknowledges that the company there had been 'a very pleasant party'.[30] He had met Miss Craik on a previous visit to Moor Park, but this was his first acquaintance with Miss Butler, and no doubt several others in the 'party'. Thus Darwin's well documented fear of new situations and encounters with strangers, was capable of being temporarily suspended and replaced by genuine conviviality.

There is another revelation in this letter relating to Darwin's supposed secrecy about his evolutionary ideas. It is apparent that Miss Butler, Miss Craik and, presumably, Darwin's other fellow diners had been treated to meal-time discourses on transmutation and the appearance of new species. Indeed, it was Georgiana Craik who had provided Darwin with an important insight into a potential pitfall of his theory. After conversations with her at Moor Park in November 1857, he had written in a geological memorandum, 'Still more why if animals have [mem. Miss Craik's objection] been modified why do we not find all intermediary fossil stages – I fully admit this one of the apparent, perhaps, real difficulties encountered, i.e. on the common view of geological record'.[31] Miss Craik's perceptive objection is all the more impressive coming from a twenty-six-year-old aspiring writer rather than a geologist or palaeontologist.[32]

It is generally claimed that Darwin withheld discussion of his theories before publication of the *Origin*, and that his thoughts on evolution were kept secret to avoid hostility and ridicule from his prejudiced contemporaries. Recent research, however, has clearly demonstrated that Darwin openly discussed transmutation with family, friends and fellow men of science during the development of his theories.[33] Darwin's letters and contemporary diaries contradict the widely held view that he kept his ideas secret because he was afraid of disapproval. The letter to Mary Butler and Darwin's earlier discussion with Georgiana Craik are wholly in keeping with this revisionist understanding of Darwin's openness, in the right company, about his views on species.

In September 1859, Darwin had written again to Mary Butler, but on this occasion the tone was pleading, not frivolous.

> My dear Miss Butler,
> My object in troubling you with this note, – a trouble, which I hope & believe you will forgive – is to know whether there is any chance of your being at Ilkley in beginning of October. It would be rather terrible to go into the great place & not know a soul. But if you were there I should feel safe and home-like. – You see that all your former kindness makes me confident of receiving more kindness.[34]

Obviously, Darwin's imploring met with a positive response and the 'nice lady' also placed herself under the care of Dr Smith at Wells House at the beginning of October that year.

Thus, Darwin's first impressions of Wells House were decidedly mixed. On the one hand the hotel seemed to be well managed, though Dr Smith lacked charisma. Darwin found him a 'sensible' but uninspiring physician, a lethargic and remote individual who was a homoeopathist to boot! For Darwin, the next few weeks under his care were going to be fraught with distrust and disbelief. But at least he had the benefit of Mary Butler's well-chosen company as he set about the major task ahead: preparing for the world's response to the publication of his revolutionary theory of the origin of species.

Notes

1   C.D. to W.D. Fox , 6 October 1859; Correspondence, 7, p. 342.

2   Anon (attributed to Nichol, J.P.), *Memorials from Ben Rhydding: Concerning the Place, its People, its Cures* (Charles Gilpin, London; James Nichol, Edinburgh: 1852).

3   The group comprised; John Crofts, Leeds, manufacturer; John Cudworth, Burley, Gentleman; William Masterman Harris, Bradford, banker; Alfred Harris the younger, Bradford, banker; Henry Rawson Morley, Leeds, iron merchant; Benjamin Briggs Popplewell, Bradford, wine merchant; George Rogers, Bradford, manufacturer. Memorial SO/199/159, West Riding Registry of Deeds, Wakefield.

4   These fields were numbered 305 and 306 on the Ilkley Tithe map, see Long, M.H., *Ilkley in 1847: An Agricultural Community on the Verge of Change* (Mid-Wharfedale Local History Research Group, Ilkley: 2005).

5   The small mill was built c. 1787 and used at various times for both cotton and worsted spinning. It was still in use for cotton spinning in 1838 but must have ceased production soon afterwards. Ingle, G., *Yorkshire Cotton: The Yorkshire Cotton Industry 1780-1835* (Carnegie Publishing, Preston: 1997) p. 219.

6   Carpenter, D., *The road to ruin: The Middeltons of Stockeld 1763-1947* (Privately published by the author, Oxford: 1999) p. 103, and Memorial SO/199/159, West Riding Registry of Deeds, Wakefield.

7   The water supply is referred to in the deeds relating to the sale of part of Ilkley Moor by the Middeltons, 8 June 1854; Memorial SO/199/159. The underground chamber was only discovered in 1973 when workmen were carrying out improvements to White Wells. *Ilkley Gazette*, 2 November 1973, p.4.

8   Linstrum, D., *West Yorkshire: Architects and Architecture* (Lund Humphries: London: 1978) p.36.

9   Brodrick went on to design several more notable buildings in Yorkshire, notably the Corn Exchange (1863) and the Mechanics Institute (1865), now the City Museum, in Leeds, and the Grand Hotel, Scarborough (1867). In 1869 at the age of forty-eight, he took up permanent residence in a suburb of Paris and abandoned architecture for a more bohemian lifestyle. See Linstrum, D., *Towers and Colonnades: The Architecture of Cuthbert Brodrick* (Leeds Philosophical and Literary Society, Leeds: 1999).

10   *Leeds Mercury*, Saturday 16 February 1856. p.6.

11   The public parks, all opened in 1846, were Queen's Park and Philips Park (in Manchester), and Peel Park (in Salford). Joshua Major was also the author of *The Theory and Practice of Landscape Gardening*, published in 1852.

12   'The New Ilkley Wells Hydropathic Establishment and Hotel'. *Leeds Mercury*, 5 June 1856, p.4.

13   Benjamin Popplewell worked in Bradford but lived at Beacon Hill in Langbar, a hamlet about five miles from Ilkley further up Wharfedale. He was a formidable, if eccentric, character. Before the railway from Bradford to Ilkley was opened in 1865 he was accustomed to walk each day from his house in Langbar to Steeton on the Keighley-Skipton line (a distance of seven miles) and catch the train into Bradford from there, repeating the journey in the evening. H. Speight, *Upper Wharfedale* (Elliot Stock, London: 1900) p.259.

14   Rischanek took up the position of Resident Physician at the newly opened Darley Dale Hydropathic Establishment, near Matlock, Derbyshire.

15   C.D. to W.D. Fox, 4 Sept 1850; Correspondence, 4, p. 354.

16   See brief obituary in *The Gentleman's Magazine*, 1864. v. 217, p. 124.

17   In 1850 Dr Smith's address was 99 Norfolk Street and in 1855 he was practicing at 6 Gell Street, both in Sheffield. See www.homeopathy.wildfalcon.com/archives/2008/08/03/edmund-smith-and-homeopathy.

18   Edmund Smith died on 5 June 1864, in Richmond, Yorkshire, aged fifty-nine. *The Gentleman's Magazine,* 1864. v. 217, p. 124.

19   *Leeds Mercury*, 1 May 1858, p.1.

20   *Leeds Mercury*, 2 November 1844, p.1.

21   The level of staffing at the hotel can be gauged from the 1861 census. At that time there were thirteen resident staff in the hotel, a 'clerk of works' resident in the porter's lodge and a gardener and his family in the other cottage. A matron lived off-site.

22   From an advertisement for a Bath Woman Attendant at Wells House, *Leeds Mercury*, 19 March 1859, p.1.

23   C.D. to John Wickham Flower, 23 March 1851; Correspondence, 5, p 8.

24   C.D. to W.D. Fox, 7 March 1852; Correspondence, 5, p.83.

25   C.D. to Daniel Sharpe, 16 October 1851; Correspondence, 5, p. 64.

26   Autobiography, p.115.

27   C.D. to Mary Butler, 20 February 1859; Correspondence, 7, p. 249.

28   Francis Darwin, Ed. *Life and Letters*, vol. 1, pp. 141-42.

29   Litchfield, H., Emma Darwin, *A Century of Family Letters 1792-1896* (John Murray, London: 1915) vol. II, p. 118.

30   C.D. to Mary Butler, 20 February 1859; Correspondence, 7, p. 249. Mary Butler was the unmarried elder sister of Richard Butler, the vicar of Trim in Co. Meath, Ireland.

31   C.D. to Emma Darwin, 28 April 1858; Correspondence, 7, p. 85, n. 4.

32   Georgiana Marion Craik (1831-95) was born in Old Brompton, London, the youngest daughter of the man of letters, George Lillie Craik (1798-1866). She began writing for *Household Words*, the weekly magazine edited by Charles Dickens, as early as 1851 (i.e. aged twenty), and published her first novel, *Riverston*, in 1857, the year she met Darwin at Moor Park. Sutherland, J., *The Stanford Companion to Victorian Fiction* (Stanford University Press, Palo Alto, CA: 1990) p.157.

33   Van Wyhe, J., 'Mind the Gap: Did Darwin avoid publishing his theory for many years?' *Notes and Records of the Royal Society*, 2007; vol. 61: 177-205.

34   C.D. to Mary Butler, 11 September 1859; Correspondence, 7, p. 331.

Chapter Two

The Lord Chancellor's Verdict

When Darwin had last seen Mary Butler, he had not yet finished writing the book setting out his theory.[1] By the time of their Ilkley rendezvous, the book, now titled *On the Origin of Species by Means of Natural Selection, or the Preservation of Favoured Races in the Struggle for Life*, was complete, with the corrected proofs in the hands of Darwin's publisher, John Murray in London. But work relating to the *Origin* continued in Ilkley. It was not incessant; indeed, Darwin at one point wrote to his friend, the botanist Joseph Hooker, that he 'cannot think how refreshing it is to idle away the whole day, & hardly ever think in the least about my confounded Book, which half killed me'. Darwin advised Hooker to follow suit, lest he one day 'stretch the string too tight'.[2] Ilkley offered opportunities for rest and amusement, and, as we shall see, Darwin took them up, as did his wife and children when they joined him. But he also engaged in regular correspondence about the *Origin*, with Murray (like many authors, Darwin made corrections up to the last minute), with Hooker and his other close scientific friends, and with important naturalists in the wider scientific community.

Darwin did not have to wait long to receive his first serious response to the book. It arrived during his first week at Wells House in the form of letters from Sir Charles Lyell, the London-based geologist and author of the famous *Principles of Geology* (1830–33). Throughout September, at Darwin's request, Murray had periodically dispatched copies of the most recently corrected batch of *Origin* proofs to Lyell. With the last batch shortly to be sent, Darwin wrote to Lyell on 30 September: 'I look at you as my Lord High Chancellor in Natural Science, & therefore… shall be deeply anxious to hear what you decide (if you are able to decide)'.[3]

In no small way, Darwin's reading of Lyell's *Principles* while on the *Beagle* in his twenties had been the making of him as a man of science. Darwin came to revere Lyell, and saw the *Origin* as extending Lyell's innovative geology – its style of reasoning as well as its understanding of earthly change – to the question of species. From Lyell, Darwin had taken over a vision of the Earth as an ancient place where wind, rain, earthquakes and other agencies operating today account for all the change there has ever been on the Earth's surface. Not for Lyell the cataclysms – such as the giant flood that supposedly bore Noah's ark – favoured by other geologists. Lyell objected that we never see such cataclysms, so should not admit them into our scientific explanations. Rather, we should restrict ourselves to the apparently humble causes that we actually observe; their effects, slowly and gradually accumulating over eons, can literally

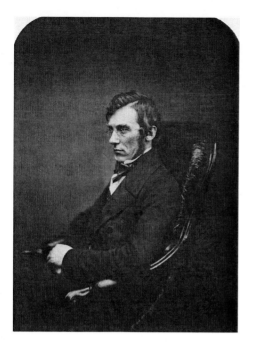

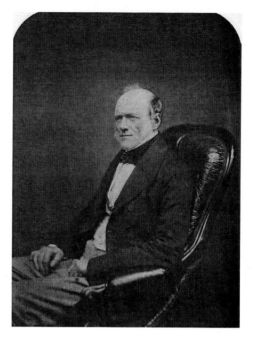

Joseph Dalton Hooker (1817-1911). A Kew-based botanist who, like Darwin, came from a distinguished scientific family but had earned a reputation in his own right through scientific voyaging as a young man – in Hooker's case, to Antarctica.
(© National Portrait Gallery, London)

Sir Charles Lyell (1797-1875). Having trained as a barrister, Lyell in his *Principles of Geology* had mounted a powerful case against the best-known transmutation theory of the early nineteenth century, due to the French naturalist Jean Baptiste de Lamarck.
(© National Portrait Gallery, London)

move mountains. Darwin became a virtuoso of Lyellian argument, and Lyell became both a trusted friend and a scientific ally. But Lyell did not believe that species evolved – or, to use the terminology of the time, that species underwent 'transmutation'. In the *Origin*, Darwin aimed to set out a case for transmutation that even Lyell would have to accept, so fully did it meet Lyell's own standards for good science.[4]

In his letter to Lyell on 30 September, Darwin had remarked that he felt convinced 'that if you are now staggered to any moderate extent' – that is, if Lyell was at all shaken in his formerly firm conviction as to the limited mutability of species – 'that you will come more & more round, the longer you keep the subject at all before your mind'.[5] And indeed Lyell had been staggered – and impressed. He delivered his initial verdict in three letters, of which two, dated 3 and 4 October, survive. 'I have just finished your volume,' Lyell wrote at the beginning of the letter of the 3rd, '& right glad I am that I did my best with Hooker to persuade you to publish… It is a splendid case of close reasoning & long sustained argument throughout'.[6] Lyell closed his letter of the 4th with the witty prediction that Darwin's book would 'form an era in geological literature'.[7] In between came a mix of editorial advice – change this word, clarify that reference, cut here, expand there, strengthen the argument as follows – and hard-hitting sceptical questioning.

Darwin's reply came in a long letter from Wells House dated 11 October. He began by thanking the older man for all the help (duly acted upon, hence at least some of the final-final corrections on the *Origin* sent from Ilkley to Murray), adding that Lyell was 'a pretty Lord Chancellor to tell the barrister on one side how best to win the cause!'[8] Although Darwin went on to address each of Lyell's numerous challenges in detail, three responses in particular merit attention here, because they deal with central features of Darwin's species theory, and because the argumentative thrust-and-parry took place at such a high level. More than anything else, the Darwin-Lyell correspondence over the *Origin* gives the lie to the notion of Darwin's Ilkley as a science-free zone.

It also usefully reminds us how intertwined were science and religion in the period. For all that Lyell wanted nothing to do with the quest for geological evidence of the Noachian flood, the divine was everywhere in his geology. In the final volume of his *Principles* he had stated that 'in whatever direction we pursue our researches, whether in time or space, we discover everywhere the clear proofs of a Creative Intelligence, and of His foresight, wisdom, and power'.[9] Journals that Lyell kept on the species question in the latter half of the 1850s show him wrestling not just with theory and evidence but with the theological implications of it all.[10] Again and again in his letters to Darwin in Ilkley, Lyell returned to the notion of species – and humans above all – as the products of a prescient, superintending intelligence. His challenges to Darwin were challenges to go further in explaining why that notion should now be dispensed with.

The first challenge to consider is raised at the beginning of Lyell's letter of the 4th. Here he touched on the very set of Galapagos Islands-related observations that had converted Darwin to the transmutation of species. Contrary to later mythology, these observations had little to do with the differences that mark out the same plant or animal groups on the different islands – the now famously varied finch beaks and so on. What mattered at the time was how similar the island-based species were to the species of the nearby South American mainland.[11]

In the *Origin*, Darwin argued that there was no way to make sense of this resemblance on the traditional, creationist view, since that view taught that different species have the distinctive forms, habits and constitutions they do because each species is designed to thrive under its particular conditions of life. Anyone taking that view might then reasonably expect that species in similar sorts of conditions will be similar, and those in very different sorts of conditions will be very different. But that is not what we find in the Galapagos-America case. Here, similar species designs serve in two very different places: the barren, rocky islands and lushly forested America. And this case was just one of many like it. Around the world, species on rocky islands resemble each other far less than they resemble species on whatever the nearby mainland is. 'I believe this grand fact can receive no sort of explanation on the ordinary view of independent creation,' wrote Darwin in the *Origin*, 'whereas on the view here maintained, it is obvious that the Galapagos Islands would be likely to receive colonists, whether by occasional means of transport or by formerly continuous land, from America; and the Cape de Verde Islands from Africa; and that such colonists would be liable to modification – the principle of inheritance still betraying their original birthplace'.[12]

The Galapagos-American story is the Darwinian evolutionary story in miniature. 'Descent with modification' was what Darwin called it: species are as they are because they are the modified descendants of nearby, previously existing species, who were themselves the modified descendants of nearby, previously existing species, who were… Map the whole set of dependencies, and you have the family tree of life – a tree growing, in Lyellian fashion, slowly and gradually, by means no different in the past from what they are in the present. To strike at the Galapagos-America example was thus to strike right at the heart of the 'one long argument' of the *Origin*. And that was just what Lyell did.

'They who never doubted about Creation,' wrote Lyell, 'can by assuming this, explain very plausibly why endemic species in the Galapagos sh[oul]d bear the stamp of the S. Ameri[ca]n type'. All these non-doubters needed to suppose, he continued, was that the Galapagos designs were future-proofed by the inclusion of features that would keep the species competitive once mainland species started arriving on the islands, as they inevitably would. Lyell explained:

> The creative power foreknows not only what range of temperature they must be prepared to withstand & what organic beings they will be in contact with for the next century but what colonists will arrive in the next 100,000 years, & as most of these will be immigrants from S. America, the same motives wh[ich] led to the endowment of the last created mollusk, fish, reptile bird or mammal with peculiar attributes on the mainland, will lead to the originating of some modification of like types for those Galapagan species which will have to struggle with the new Colonists, so that even were there no inorganic conditions, common to the Galapagos & S. America, or common to Africa & other regions, which is very improbable, there w[oul]d still be reasons why the new insular species sh[oul]d be gifted with S American characters. Without these they will not last.[13]

Especially galling to Darwin, one imagines, was the way the argument made use of a principle that the *Origin* insisted on over and over again: that relations among species are far more important than the relations each has to the physical environment in determining the forms of species.[14] But by the time Darwin put pen to paper, he had his answer: 'I cannot agree with you that [Galapagos] species if created to struggle with American forms would have to be created on the American type. Facts point diametrically the other way'. One such fact was that European plants, so different from the American ones, had dominated wherever introduced in Argentina. Darwin saw in this phenomenon the workings of a more general rule: the plants and animals that thrive in a new place, enough to become 'naturalised', tend to come from somewhere very different, and accordingly to have very different designs. In that light, Lyell's 'creative power', if it had acted with the acute foreknowledge that Lyell ascribed, would surely have created the Galapagos species to something other than the American type, the better to ensure their long-term survival over American interlopers.[15]

Lyell mounted a second but similarly directed attack over the question of organs that, like male nipples (to cite one of Darwin's examples in the *Origin*), are so rudimentary as to be useless. Not, one might think, very good design principles at work there! And indeed, as Darwin emphasised, the independent creation view struggled to explain such organs, supposing them to lend pleasing symmetry to the overall organisational plan to which the creative power worked. Darwin reckoned that his proposal about the genealogical connectedness of species made much more sense of the problem. Rudimentary organs exist, Darwin argued, because the organisms sporting them are descended from species in which the organs were well-developed. Under the ancestors' conditions, the organs were useful. Under the descendants', they are useless, and the organs have accordingly become diminished.[16]

But Lyell was unmoved. Once again, he flagged the possibility that Darwin had neglected the creative power's capacity for foreknowledge – in this case, of what the descendants of the rudimentary-organ bearers will need. A scientific friend, Lyell wrote, had 'once suggested to me that rudimentary organs may be quite as often the germs of organs about to be enjoyed by descendants as the remains of organs bec[o]me abortive. What say you to this?' One should not be tempted, Lyell subsequently made plain, to dismiss the question as unanswerable on the grounds that we cannot know for certain what will happen in the future. For, of course, what is now present had once been future; so one may ask whether certain now well-developed organs can be traced back to primordia that, examined in isolation, look for all the world like useless rudiments. 'Before an Apteryx' – a flightless bird – 'can grow into a flying bird must there not be thousands of generations with rudimentary wings? In that case instead of the rudiment being genealogical, it becomes as Agassiz [the Swiss-American creationist naturalist Louis Agassiz] might say prophetic'.[17]

Nothing could have been more remote from the vision of life put forward in the *Origin*. For Darwin, species turn out as they do not because of any planning or superintendence, but because ancestral species happen to find themselves in certain kinds of new environments, and to become modified in certain ways. And that is it. In taking up Lyell's challenge, Darwin introduced a distinction, between 'nascent' organs, which are useful and on their way in, and 'rudimentary' organs, which are useless and on their way out. How to tell the difference between them, given that it can be hard to rule out total uselessness or minimal usefulness? Go to history, Darwin suggested. Nascent organs will likely not go back very far, wrote Darwin, 'for beings with any important organ but little developed will generally have been supplanted by their descendants with the organs well developed'. Rudimentary organs, by contrast, will go back a long way. Darwin returned to an example he had used in the *Origin*: the bastard wing – a small, feather-covered digit on the front edge of the wings of modern birds. 'The bastard-wing of birds is rudimentary digit,' wrote Darwin, '& I believe that if ever fossil birds are found very low down in series, they will be seen to have a double or bifurcated wing. Here is a bold prophecy! To admit prophetic germs is tantamount to rejecting theory of Natural Selection'.[18]

Natural selection was Darwin's theory of the main process driving genealogical species change. For all Lyell's hesitancy, this theory too is profoundly Lyellian. It tells of how small-scale causes in observable operation today have, by the slow, gradual accumulation of their effects, brought about changes so impressive that the ignorant are tempted to ascribe them to miracles. One such cause is the regular production of offspring who inherit some of their parents' traits, including traits that, in some small way, make them better at the business of surviving and reproducing than other individuals of the same species. Another is the regular overproduction of such offspring, which means that there is always a terrible struggle to survive long enough to reproduce. Add these causes together in the mind, as Darwin asked readers of the *Origin* to do, and you will see that in every generation there is a natural sorting, or selection, in favour of those individuals who happen to be born with traits – greater speed, greater intelligence, whatever it might be – that make for a competitive edge. And as this selection process repeats itself down the generations, the average species type gradually changes, becoming ever more perfectly adapted to local conditions. At the limit, the species looks as if designed for those conditions. But there was never any foresight involved – no purposeful, guided directedness toward a goal. At every stage, what was preserved in the struggle was what was useful then and there. As Darwin emphasised in his letter to Lyell, 'Natural Selection acts exclusively by preserving successive slight, useful modifications, hence nat. select. cannot possibly make a *useless* or rudimentary organ'.[19]

Natural selection was more directly at issue in the third exchange to be considered here, over the origin of humankind, or 'Man', as the Victorians had it. Much to Darwin's satisfaction, Lyell would soon accept the Darwinian theory as applicable for all species except – much to Darwin's annoyance – Man. In Lyell's letter of the 4th, he signalled just how hard he found it to suppose that natural selection could possibly have wrought man from nonhuman starting materials. In this matter, Lyell was prepared to side with the cataclysm mongers. Is not, Lyell asked, 'Man's appearance in the organic what a cataclysm w[oul]d be in the inorganic world. What c[oul]d Selection do in adding new powers, attributes & forces, were not a creative power assumed as part of the reproductive or variety[-]making natural law'. Lyell went on to issue his most wounding judgement:

> This theory cannot I fear compare scientifically to the *verae causae* [true, real causes, whose existence is not merely hypothetical but witnessed] to which you & I now refer the inorganic changes. It resembles more the inventions of the old cosmogonists for altho' it assumes that all this machinery is now going on & at work & that the changes are not brought about by extinct or unknown causes, yet the power which can superinduce the intelligence of the Elephant into a planet which had nothing above that of a fish at an earlier period & then produce Man in his highest state is not a comprehensible *vera causa* – or one the mode of working of which we can hope to understand.[20]

On the matter of whether natural selection would have needed 'new powers, attributes & forces' to bring Man into being, Darwin's reply was robust. As long as one allows that intellect is useful, and that some individuals are endowed with more of it than others, natural selection theory can handily explain the evolution of greater intelligence. Darwin wrote to Lyell:

> I suppose that you do not doubt that the intellectual powers are as important for the welfare of each being, as corporeal structure: if so, I can see no difficulty in the most intellectual individuals of a species being continually selected; & the intellect of the new species thus improved... I look at this process as now going on with the races of man; the less intellectual races being exterminated... I would give absolutely nothing for theory of nat. selection, if it requires miraculous additions at any one stage of descent... I think you will be driven to reject all or admit all: I fear by your letter it will be the former alternative; & in that case I shall feel sure it is my fault & not the theory's fault, & this will certainly comfort me.[21]

It is jarring to imagine Darwin at his desk, in the splendour of his rooms at Wells House, amid the peaceful surroundings of the sheep-dotted slopes of Ilkley Moor, conjuring a vision of imperial race war. Equally jarring is to consider that, while he was working out his multiple and complex rebuttals of Lyell's criticisms, undertaking mental travel back to the Galapagos Islands and deep into the rocks where fossil birds might be found, the state of his body was his major preoccupation. Darwin had come to Ilkley in search of relief from debilitating illness. For the next weeks, and for all that the *Origin* would regularly ensnare him, he would lead the life of a devotee of the Ilkley water cure.

Notes

1   Darwin's gradual progress on the *Origin* throughout 1858 and 1859 can be tracked in his 'Journal', as transcribed in Appendix II, Correspondence, 7, pp. 503–504.

2   C.D. to J.D. Hooker, 15 October [1859]; Correspondence, 7, p. 350.

3   C.D. to Charles Lyell, 30 September [1859]; Correspondence, 7, p. 338. On Lyell's reading of the *Origin* through September, see footnote 2, Correspondence, 7, p. 342.

4   On Darwin's debt to Lyell, see Hodge, J. and Radick, G. (eds), *The Cambridge Companion to Darwin*, 2nd edition (Cambridge University Press, Cambridge 2009), chs 1 & 2.

5   C.D. to Charles Lyell, 30 September [1859]; Correspondence, 7, p. 338.

6   Charles Lyell to C.D., 3 October 1859; Correspondence, 7, pp. 339–340. Darwin wrote to Hooker on 15 October: 'Lyell has been *extremely* kind in writing me three volume-like letters'. C.D. to J.D. Hooker, 15 October 1859; Correspondence, 7, p. 349, emphasis in original.

7   Charles Lyell to C.D., 4 October 1859; Correspondence, 13, p. 414.

8   C.D. to Charles Lyell, 11 October [1859]; Correspondence, 7, p. 343. For some of the changes that Darwin made to the *Origin* in the light of Lyell's suggestions, see footnotes 7 and 9, Correspondence, 7, p. 342.

9   Lyell, C., *Principles of Geology* (Penguin, London 1997), p. 437.

10   Wilson, L.G. (ed.), *Sir Charles Lyell's Scientific Journals on the Species Question* (Yale University Press, New Haven and London 1970).

11   On the significance of the Galapagos for Darwin, see Hodge, J., 'The notebook programmes and projects of Darwin's London years', in Hodge, J., and Radick, G. (eds), *The Cambridge Companion to Darwin*, 2nd edition (Cambridge University Press, Cambridge 2009), pp. 47–48.

12   Darwin, C., *On the Origin of Species* (John Murray, London 1859), pp. 398–399.

13   Charles Lyell to C.D., 4 October 1859; Correspondence, 13, p. 411. Here Lyell rang changes on a familiar theme in his geology; see Lyell, C., *Principles of Geology* (Penguin, London 1997), p. 200.

14   See, e.g., Darwin, C., *On the Origin of Species* (John Murray, London 1859), pp. 60, 77–78.

15   C.D. to Charles Lyell, 11 October [1859]; Correspondence, 7, p. 343. Apparently this response went deep with Lyell. Years later, he told his friend Charles Bunbury that, as Bunbury recalled, 'nothing contributed more to shake [Lyell's] belief in the old doctrine (which he formerly held) of the independent creation of species, than the facts of which so many have lately been recorded, relating to the rapid naturalization of certain plants in countries newly colonized by Europeans'. Quoted in Hodge, J., 'Darwin's reception in England', *Darwin Studies: A Theorist and His Theories in Their Contexts* (Ashgate, Farnham 2009), VIII, p. 29. We are grateful to Jon Hodge for drawing this passage to our attention.

16   Darwin, C., *On the Origin of Species* (John Murray, London 1859), pp. 450–456.

17   Charles Lyell to C.D., 4 October 1859; Correspondence, 13, p. 414.

18   C.D. to Charles Lyell, 11 October [1859]; Correspondence, 7, pp. 346–347. The distinction between rudimentary and nascent organs was one of the few additions to the *Origin* that Darwin introduced for the second edition; Correspondance, 7, p. 411, footnote 4.

19   C.D. to Charles Lyell, 11 October [1859]; Correspondence, 7, p. 347, emphasis in original.

20   Charles Lyell to C.D., 4 October 1859; Correspondence, 13, pp. 411–412.

21   C.D. to Charles Lyell, 11 October [1859]; Correspondence, 7, p. 345.

Chapter Three

Illness and the Water Cure

In the same letter to Fox asking whether he too might join Darwin in Ilkley, Darwin had added:

> I came here intending to stay for 3 or 4 weeks, but I very much doubt whether I shall have patience. – But this morning's post has brought me note from Emma telling me to look out for a House, as she is greatly inclined to come here. But I have not least idea whether there is a House which would suit or how I could do my water-cure out of Establishment. – So everything is utterly uncertain. I heartily wish you would come, but I dare not advise or press it.[1]

Darwin began to make enquiries about accommodation for himself and his family. In the meantime, he entered into the daily routine at Wells House, determined to make the most of the treatments on offer, even if they were prescribed by a physician in whom he had little confidence.

Naturally, the most important aspect of the daily routine was the bath (or baths) prescribed by Dr Smith. Hydropathic physicians had several ways of delivering the cold-water cure to their patients; in Dr Smith's case wet-sheeting was the mainstay of treatment. Darwin had endured wet-sheets before, so he was completely familiar with this particular kind of water-torture. It began with the bath-attendant immersing linen sheets in buckets of cold water while the patient stripped down to a pair of calico drawers. The attendant wrung out the sheets to remove excess water but left them thoroughly damp, then encircled the patient with the partly folded sheets. In this way, two or three sheets swathed the torso and upper legs, leaving the arms and lower legs free, to allow some movement. For even greater effect a small wet towel could be applied to the head like a large damp turban. Thus encumbered, the patient was left in a lying position, or put in a plain wooden seat, or allowed to walk around the treatment rooms. The sheets remained in place for up to two or three hours. As every student of elementary physics is aware, evaporation leads to cooling, and under the sheets the body surface underwent a slow and progressive reduction in temperature. When the requisite time had passed, the patient was divested of the dreaded sheets and given a brisk rub-down with soft towels. Then, blessed relief, the patient experienced the sought-for 'reaction'. In the 'reaction' phase, the contracted blood vessels in the skin underwent sudden dilatation with a rebound increase in blood–flow, and blood at normal body temperature now reached the extremities. The grateful patient felt the ruddy glow of health – a feeling of heat where formerly there was cold and numbness – warmth and relief that in the patient's mind attested to the powerful therapeutic effects of the cold water application.

Dr Smith had many other treatments in his armamentarium. Sometimes he advocated a straightforward cold-water plunge bath, but more often water was delivered as a douche; as a drizzle or needle shower; or a spinal, head, foot or Sitz bath. The latter was a particular favourite. Naked apart from dry towels around the shoulders and upper body, the patient climbed into the bath and sat on a perforated seat. The 'seat' was the entry point for water poured into the connecting U-tube by the bath-attendant. Thus the bath would be filled with cold-water that had emerged around the patient's fundament. Water was added until the level in the bath covered the hips ('shallow Sitz') or up to mid-chest level ('deep Sitz'). Ten to twenty minutes sitting in cold water was a reliable cure for constipation. Perhaps the bath's popularity owed something to the diet at Wells House.

Dr Smith held firmly to the opinion that indiscriminate eating and drinking was injurious to health. Another visitor to Wells House recorded his opinions of the hydropathic diet:

In chronic complaints especially, dietetic indulgence is slow suicide.[2] Every year, hundreds and thousands of highly-respectable people kill themselves with their knives and forks. Hydropathy sees the evil of complicated food, and regulates its diet tables with studious simplicity. White and brown bread, plain or toasted, fresh butter, and lightly-boiled eggs, constitute the water-patients' breakfast. His thirst he quenches with water, milk, cocoa, or black tea. At dinner he may cut and come again at beef, mutton, fowl, and vegetables, preceded occasionally by white fish, and followed invariably by plain puddings and stewed fruit. Bread and the necessary condiments are allowed in moderation; and water is, of course, the only beverage. Whatever is placed before the water patient is pure and good, which, cannot often be said of the made-up dishes and loaded wines of the

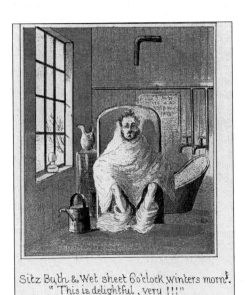

Sitz Bath & Wet sheet 6o'clock winters morn.̃ "This is delightful, very !!!"

Wet-sheeting was the mainstay of Dr Smith's hydropathic regime. Here it is combined with a Sitz bath, a formidable dual treatment.

purple and apoplectic bon vivant. The pure, clear, and sparkling liquid that gushes from the Ilkley hills is not less exhilarating, and is much more wholesome, than manufactured champagne. And of such water, may be said with truth, what is falsely said of such wine, that there "is not a headache in a hogshead of it." After a hydropathic meal there is no indigestion, no nightmare, no headache next morning, no sickness next day. The body feels light and the head clear; and the general feeling is the satisfaction of a rational being who has eaten enough for the support of the body, not the bloated sensation of a prize-pig.

Such was the plain and substantial fare on offer to Charles Darwin as he underwent the water cure – and the whole regime seemed to suit him. A few days after sending off his letter to Lyell, Darwin wrote to his botanist friend Hooker:

> I have been here nearly a fortnight, & it has done me very much good; ... Before starting here I was in an awful state of stomach, strength, temper & spirits... You cannot think how refreshing it is to idle away whole day & hardly ever think in the least about my confounded Book, which half killed me. If I could keep at home like I feel here, I shd be a man again; & should so enjoy a little society of my friends.[3]

How can this remarkable recovery be explained? What was the 'scientific' basis of the water cure and why had Darwin become convinced by its healing properties?

By October 1859, Darwin had suffered ill health for over twenty-two years. It was in 1837, a year after returning to England from his voyage on the *Beagle*, that he first acknowledged he had a persistent health problem. In a letter to his old Cambridge tutor, Professor Henslow, Darwin admits, 'I have not been very well of late with an uncomfortable palpitation of the heart, and my doctors urge me strongly to knock off all work & go and live in the country for a few weeks. I believe I must do this'.[4]

Not that palpitation was his only health problem. Darwin's illness was dominated by 'fits' of vomiting, but he also suffered from intermittent abdominal pain, skin rashes that he termed 'eczema', 'erythema' or 'eruptions', tiredness and lethargy, headaches and a multitude of other less-frequent complaints. These symptoms varied in their severity, but he was rarely free of one complaint or another. His illness appears to have fluctuated according to stressful events. He was particularly bad in the early years of his marriage (from 1839-44), although in choosing to marry his cousin, Emma Wedgwood, Darwin found the perfect 'nurse' and comforter. Nevertheless, it was a period of anxiety as he wrestled with the competing demands of wife and children (William Erasmus, born December 1839; Anne Elizabeth ('Annie'), born March 1841; Mary Eleanor, born September 1842 but died a few weeks later; Henrietta Emma ('Etty'), born September 1843), and his all-consuming researches and writing. It was during this period, that along with his account of the *Beagle* voyage, he wrote his five evolutionary notebooks culminating in 1844 in his first 'sketch' of the species problem with its revolutionary ideas on transmutation.

Naturally, Darwin sought medical advice for his intractable illness. His first port of call was his father, Dr Robert Waring Darwin, a well-respected and successful general practitioner in Shrewsbury. Indeed, it was through their frequent communications about the course of his illness that Charles and his father established a close personal relationship.[5] Until his death in

1848, Dr Darwin regularly gave Charles prescriptions in response to the latest exacerbation of his symptoms. For example, in November 1840 Dr Darwin prescribed logwood (used for diarrhoea), cinnamon (to improve appetite and digestion) and potassium bicarbonate (an alkali, to counteract gastric acidity).[6] As with most new treatments, Darwin experienced some short-lived benefit, but then his symptoms returned to their former severity. Darwin also consulted some of the foremost medical men of the day. Early in his illness, he saw the eminent physician Dr Henry Holland, a distant cousin of the Darwins and Wedgwoods, who was baffled by Darwin's protean symptoms and whose treatments were ineffective. Darwin also consulted Dr James Clark, physician-in-ordinary to Queen Victoria, who claimed that a permanent move from London into the country might ameliorate Darwin's dyspepsia. This advice prompted the purchase of Down House, near Bromley in Kent.

Robert Darwin, and the other physicians that Charles consulted, prescribed numerous medicaments that were of dubious efficacy and, in some instances, potentially harmful. For his stomach complaints he was given bitters and tonics, bismuth, mineral acids, alkalies, pepsin, 'Condy's Ozonised Water' and phosphate of iron[7] while arsenic solution, tartar emetic ointment and Mr Startin's 'muddy stuff' were applied to his eczematous skin.[8] None of these treatments, however, achieved more than a transient improvement in his symptoms. Darwin's eagerness to try new treatments was born more out of desperation than confidence in their potential efficacy, but gradually his faith in pills and potions waned and he became more receptive to alternative, nature-centred approaches. Such an approach was suggested to him in 1848.

In the years immediately before, Darwin had been busy with *Geological Observations on South America* and a book on barnacles. More children had arrived – George Howard in July 1845 and Elizabeth (Lizzy) in July 1847, to add to their three surviving children. As the family increased so Darwin had become more anxious about hereditary disease, a fear not helped by the early death of Mary Eleanor. Although a marriage between cousins was commonplace, particularly among the Wedgwood dynasty, Darwin began to suspect that his children were affected by 'the worst of my bugbears, hereditary weakness' as a result of his marriage to Emma.[9] To add to his anxieties, he became increasingly concerned for his father's health. He was very dependent upon his father, not only for medical advice, but also for financial support. Darwin's own health deteriorated and he complained of recurrent vomiting, sudden shivering attacks and weakness.[10] Another child (Francis) was born in August 1848, and over the summer months Emma would not have been able to give Charles the 'nursing' he thought his condition merited.

In the autumn of 1848, Darwin was visited by an old *Beagle* shipmate, Bartholomew Sulivan, who found him weak and in low spirits. Sulivan suggested that Darwin should undertake a course of hydropathy, and recommended Dr James Gully of Malvern. Sulivan assured him that Gully's treatment had benefited many people with similar dyspectic diseases. The suggestion was met with scepticism; nevertheless Darwin resolved to pursue the matter. He consulted his father, who recommended that he should try it when the weather turned warmer, in the spring. But this proved to be the last medical advice he gave to his son. Dr Robert Darwin died on 13 November 1848, and it was a measure of Charles Darwin's poor state of health that he declared himself unable to attend his father's funeral or to act as one of his executors.[11]

The next three months were spent in grieving (and guilt), and in sporadic work on the barnacles. He continued to be severely ill, and early in February 1849, his cousin Fox urged him to try the water cure, but Darwin remained reluctant. Nevertheless, he determined to get

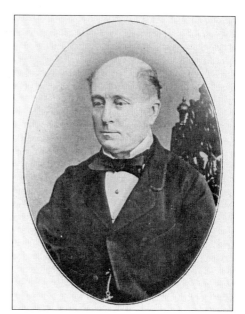

Dr James Manby Gully (1808-83). Along with Dr James Wilson, Gully was responsible for introducing the water cure into Britain. 'I like Dr Gully very much,' wrote Darwin, '– he is certainly an able man He is very kind & attentive; but seems puzzled with my case'.

a copy of Gully's book.[12] By the end of February, however, he had 'resolved to go this early summer & spend two months at Malvern & see whether there is any truth in Gully & the water cure: regular Doctors cannot check my incessant vomiting at all'.[13] Obviously, Gully's book had aroused Darwin's curiosity and expectations to a level that persuaded him to 'take the plunge' and visit Malvern.[14]

The concept of 'the water cure' has to be distinguished from the long-established practice of 'taking the waters'. People 'took the waters' at spas where particular springs had been identified whose waters were credited with medicinal properties. Thus, places like Bath, Cheltenham and Tunbridge Wells in the South; Droitwich, Leamington and Woodhall Spa in the Midlands; and Buxton and Harrogate in the North of England, offered 'healing waters' from their chalybeate springs; together with baths (usually warm), massage, wax treatments, and diverse entertainments, all provided in an atmosphere of gentility, refinement and luxury.[15] 'The water cure' by contrast, was a system of treatment involving the application of cold water (preferably ice-cold water) by way of baths, douches or wet-sheets, combined with drinking copious quantities of pure water to 'flush out' accumulated waste products, together with regular exercise, dietary restrictions and temperance. This disciplined regime contrasted markedly with the attractions, diversions and intemperance found in the existing spas and provided an opportunity for new, 'hydropathic' resorts to be established, as at Malvern and Ilkley, where rigour, routine and self-denial were the watch-words.

The water cure was developed, if not exactly discovered, in the 1820s by Vinzenz (Vincent) Priessnitz (1799-1851), the semi-literate son of a peasant farmer in the village of Gräfenberg in Silesia (now the Czech Republic).[16] During the 1830s, news of the 'Gräfenberg treatment' and its many 'cures' spread throughout Europe. Visitors flocked to Priessnitz's establishment in ever-increasing numbers. In 1842, two Englishmen who would be instrumental in the introduction of hydrotherapy into this country visited Gräfenberg: Dr James Wilson, a general

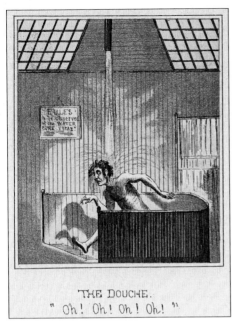

THE DOUCHE.
" Oh! Oh! Oh! Oh! "

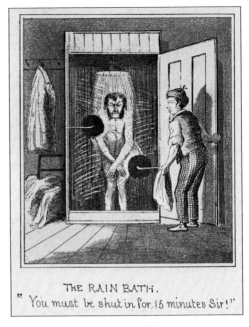

THE RAIN BATH.
" You must be shut in for 15 minutes Sir!"

On occasions, Dr Smith prescribed a douche as a way of delivering the cold water…

… at other times he favoured the drizzle or needle bath.

practitioner from Clapton, in the east end of London, who established the water cure in Malvern; and a Leeds businessman, Hamer Stansfeld, who was responsible for its foundation in Ilkley. After several weeks' hydropathic treatment in Gräfenberg, both men returned to England with their health restored.

On his return to London, Wilson, now a zealous disciple of Priessnitz and his methods, persuaded a medical friend with a practice in the fashionable west end of London, James Manby Gully, to join him in founding a hydropathic practice. After researching several possible locations, they selected the Worcestershire town of Malvern – a place chosen for its pure water, upland air and the opportunities provided by the Malvern Hills for healthy exercise. In July 1842, Wilson took a lease on an inn in the town, and renamed it 'Gräfenberg House'. Gully moved to Malvern three months later having purchased two houses, one to be used as a family residence, and the other to accommodate patients. After a few years of cooperation, however, the Wilson-Gully partnership ran into difficulties. Wilson decided to erect a purpose-built hydropathic establishment for his own use, and his 'Priessnitz House' was completed in 1845. In 1846, Gully published his influential book, *The Water Cure in Chronic Disease*, a best-seller of its day. In a footnote, Gully was openly critical of Wilson and his encouragement of patients to publish quasi-medical works that gave an inaccurate, if glowing, account of the water cure. This public rebuke must have marked the final act in their declining relationship. When Gully moved his family home to the town centre in 1847, he was able to use his two adjacent houses to accommodate male and female patients separately as, unlike Dr Wilson, he thought it undesirable to mix the sexes when they were undergoing treatment. The two buildings were joined by a short covered bridge, somewhat unoriginally called the 'Bridge of Sighs'.[17]

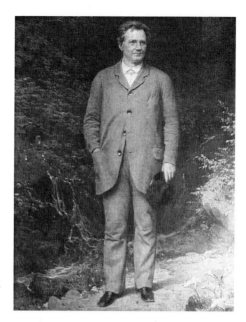

Vinzenz (Vincent) Priessnitz (1799-1851), discoverer of the water cure. (By permission of Petr Neugebauer)

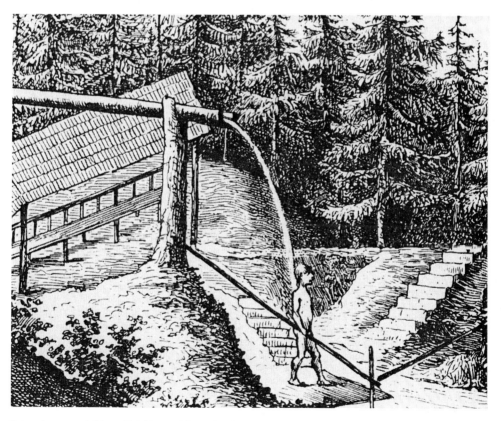

Priessnitz created this artificial 'waterfall' or douche at his establishment in Gräfenberg. This treatment was considered most efficacious in cases of lumbago or sciatica. (Petr Neugebauer)

THE

WATER CURE

IN

CHRONIC DISEASE:

An Exposition

OF THE CAUSES, PROGRESS, AND TERMINATIONS OF VARIOUS
CHRONIC DISEASES OF THE DIGESTIVE ORGANS,
LUNGS, NERVES, LIMBS, AND SKIN;
AND OF THEIR TREATMENT BY WATER,
AND OTHER HYGIENIC MEANS.

BY

JAMES MANBY GULLY, M.D.

LICENTIATE OF THE ROYAL COLLEGE OF SURGEONS,
AND FELLOW OF THE ROYAL PHYSICAL SOCIETY, EDINBURGH;
FELLOW OF THE ROYAL MEDICAL AND CHIRURGICAL
SOCIETY, LONDON, ETC.

NINTH EDITION.

LONDON:
SIMPKIN, MARSHALL, & CO., PATERNOSTER ROW
EDINBURGH: A. C. BLACK. MALVERN: HENRY LAMB;
AND AT THE RAILWAY STATIONS.
1863.

Left: Title page of *The Water Cure in Chronic Disease* – the book that persuaded Darwin of the efficacy of hydropathy and prompted his visit to Malvern. Gully's book was first published in 1846 and proved to be highly popular, running to several editions.

Below: Priessnitz placed great emphasis on physical exercise as an adjunct to the water treatment. Thus, strenuous walks in the hills around Gräfenberg were considered obligatory. If the weather was inclement however, he adopted some novel approaches. Here, a lady patient is sawing a log in her bedroom, having discarded the Indian clubs and the dumb-bells! (Petr Neugebauer)

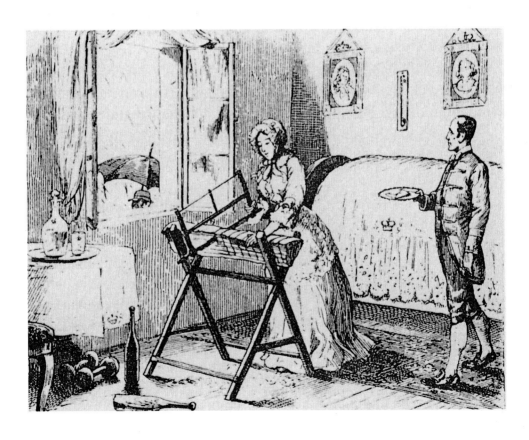

Over the ensuing years Dr Gully's reputation flourished, and he built-up a lucrative practice. This owed more to his personal charm than the success rate of his treatments, but there is no doubt that many patients benefited from one or more aspects of his regime. Whether or not it was the cold-water treatment *per se* is open to question. Whatever the explanation, more and more patients were attracted to Malvern and to Dr Gully, including a number of celebrities, among them Alfred, Lord Tennyson (who first visited in 1847) and Florence Nightingale (1848). The latter attested to Gully's charm when, after taking her mother for a consultation, she wrote: 'Mama was so taken in by him that I was obliged to tell him that I had a father living'.[18] By the 1850s it was estimated, at least by his envious rivals, that Gully was earning £10,000 per annum – an enormous income at that time, worth around a million pounds in today's values.[19]

Darwin travelled to Malvern in March 1849 accompanied by his wife, six children, Joseph Parslow (their faithful butler), a governess, and maids. He rented a villa – an arrangement that allowed Darwin to escape some of the more troublesome restrictions of the water cure regime, such as the writing of letters (which Gully frowned upon as it taxed the brain), and the ban on taking snuff, one of Darwin's favourite 'little pleasures'. His initial consultation with Gully proved to be a positive experience. Darwin declared, 'I like Dr Gully very much – he is certainly an able man… He is very kind & attentive; but seems puzzled with my case – thinks my head or top of spinal chord cause of mischief'.[20] It appears from this comment, and from the treatment regime that Gully prescribed for Darwin, that he considered him to have a form of 'nervous dyspepsia', a condition caused by 'the close application of the mind to any one subject' and resulting in congestion of the blood vessels in the stomach. Gully postulated that disease in the stomach had repercussions on the rest of the body. A malfunctioning stomach made 'bad' blood which had an adverse effect on other organs and caused systemic disease. He further claimed that the external application of cold water counteracted this congestion

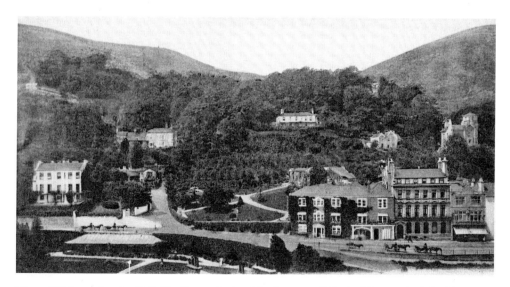

View of Malvern showing Belle Vue Terrace in the right foreground. The building on the left of this terrace was the Crown Inn. The inn was purchased by Dr James Wilson in 1842 and converted into a hydropathic establishment – the first in the British Isles. Appropriately, he re-named it 'Gräfenberg House'.

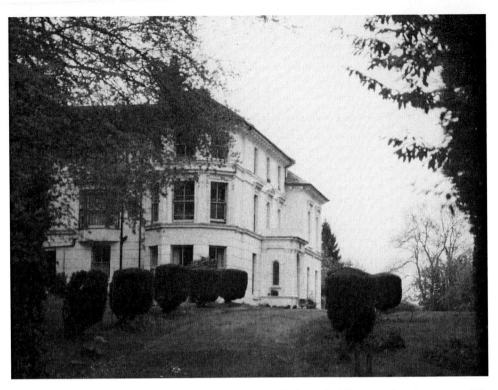

The Lodge, Worcester Road, Great Malvern. Darwin rented 'The Lodge' from March to June 1849 while he was undergoing treatment in Malvern. The handsome villa was required to accommodate his family (Emma and six children), the butler, a governess, and maids.

by stimulating ganglionic nerves in the skin whose signals, modulated through the brain and spinal cord, brought about a contraction of the blood vessels around the stomach. Restricted blood flow to the stomach in turn lessened the morbid 'inflammatory' processes that led to its malfunction.[21]

Having digested Gully's explanations, Darwin embarked on his watery path to health with great enthusiasm and confidence. He gave a full account of the treatment in a letter to his sister Susan in which he described his daily routine:

1/4 before 7. get up, & am scrubbed with rough towel in cold water for 2 or 3 minutes, which after the few first days, made & makes me very like a lobster— I have a washerman, a very nice person, & he scrubs behind, whilst I scrub in front.— drink a tumbler of water & get my clothes on as quick as possible & walk for 20 minutes— I cd. walk further, but I find it tires me afterwards— I like all this very much.— At same time I put on a compress, which is a broad wet folded linen covered by mackintosh & which is "refreshed"—ie dipt in cold water every 2 hours & I wear it all day, except for about 2 hours after midday dinner; I don't perceive much effect from this of any kind.— After my walk, shave & wash & get my breakfast, which was to have been exclusively toast with meat or egg, but he has allowed me a little milk to sop the stale toast in. At no time must I take any sugar, butter, spices tea bacon or anything good.— At 12 oclock I put my feet for 10 minutes in cold water with a little mustard & they are violently rubbed by my man; the coldness makes my feet ache much, but upon the whole my feet are certainly less cold than formerly.— Walk for 20 minutes & dine at one.— He has relaxed a little about my dinner & says I may try plain pudding, if I am sure it lessens sickness.— After dinner lie down & try to go to sleep for one hour.— At 5 oclock feet in cold water—drink cold water & walk as before— Supper same as breakfast at 6 oclock.— I have had much sickness this week, but certainly I have felt much stronger & the sickness has depressed me much less.— Tomorrow I am to be packed at 6 oclock A.M for 1 & 1/2 hour in Blanket, with hot bottle to my feet & then rubbed with cold dripping sheet; but I do not know anything about this.[20]

Gradually, the sickness diminished and Darwin began to feel restored.

After a stay of four months, Darwin and his entourage returned to Down on 30 June. He resolved to carry on the water treatment, even to the extent of building a douche in the grounds. 'I consider the sickness as absolutely cured,' Darwin declared. 'The Water Cure is assuredly a grand discovery & how sorry I am I did not hear of it, or rather that I was not compelled to try it some five or six years ago'.[22] He kept up the treatment at home for two years, writing regular reports to Dr Gully who in turn 'instructed' him on any modifications to the regime.[23] In March 1851, however, he returned to Malvern, not on this occasion because of a relapse in his own symptoms, but in a desperate bid to restore the health of his daughter, Annie.

In the summer of 1850, when Annie was nine years old, her health 'began to break down'.[24] The family, now including baby Leonard ('Lennie'), born January 1850, went to Ramsgate

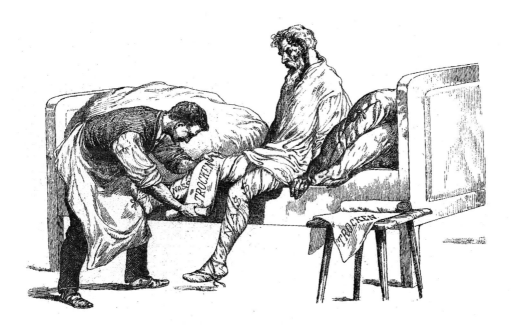

Wrapping patients in wet sheets was of general utility in achieving the 'cure by cold-water'. Here, the wet sheets ('nass') are enclosed in a layer of dry ('trocken') sheets to hold in the moisture. (Petr Neugebauer)

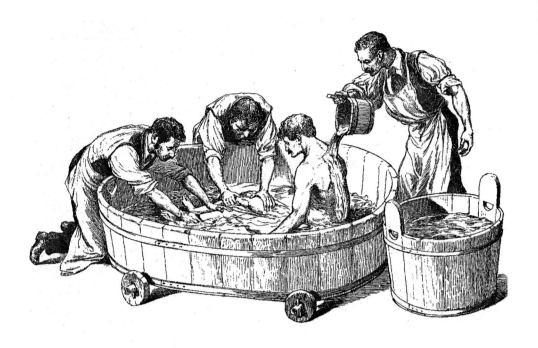

Priessnitz improvised cold-water baths from giant wine butts. Here bathing is combined with massage and continuous drenching of the patient's back with cold water. (Petr Neugebauer)

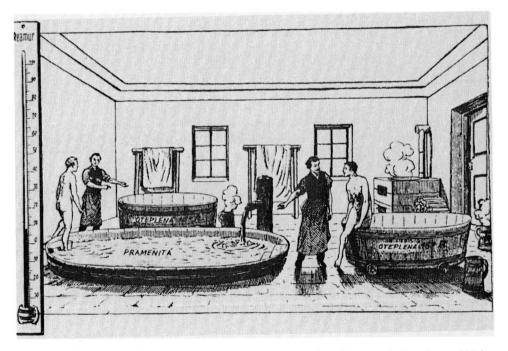

In a departure from the pure cold-water regime, these patients endure alternating baths at low and high temperature. (Petr Neugebauer)

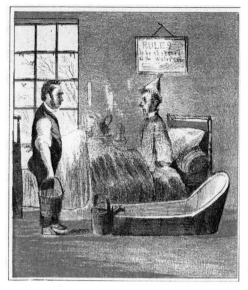

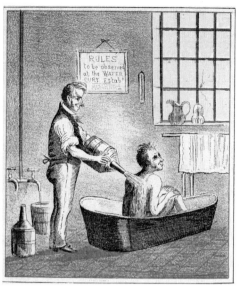

Darwin gives a detailed account of his treatment at Malvern: '1/4 before 7. get up, & am scrubbed with rough towel in cold water for 2 or 3 minutes, which after the few first days, made & makes me very like a lobster'.

'I have a washerman, a very nice person, & he scrubs behind, whilst I scrub in front'.

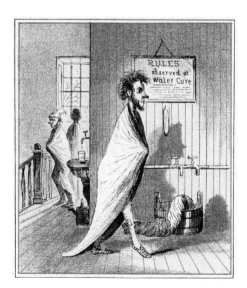

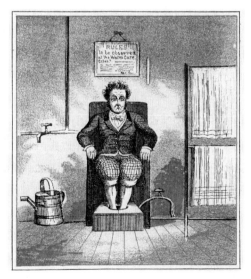

'At same time I put on a compress, which is a broad wet folded linen covered by mackintosh & which is "refreshed"—ie dipt in cold water every 2 hours & I wear it all day, except for about 2 hours after midday dinner; I don't perceive much effect from this of any kind'.

'At 12 oclock I put my feet for 10 minutes in cold water with a little mustard & they are violently rubbed by my man; the coldness makes my feet ache much, but upon the whole my feet are certainly less cold than formerly'.

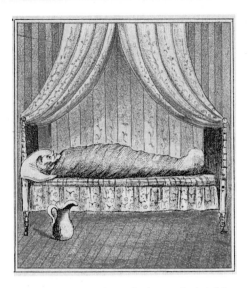

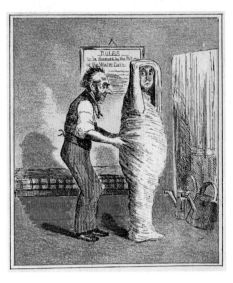

'Tomorrow I am to be packed at 6 oclock A.M for 1 & 1/2 hour in Blanket, with hot bottle to my feet…'

'…& then rubbed with cold dripping sheet; but I do not know anything about this'.

in October 'on her account, but with no success'. Faced with her continuing deterioration, Darwin took Annie to Malvern on 24 March 1851 and placed her under the care of Dr Gully. Annie's sister, Henrietta, went along as a companion; their old nurse, Brodie, and Miss Thorley, the governess, were left in charge when Darwin returned (via a short stay in London) to Down. Emma could not go to Malvern as she was 'expecting to be confined in May' (another son, Horace, was born on 13 May). On 17 April, Darwin was summoned to Malvern and found Annie hardly recognizable in her wasted, terminal condition. He spent the following days in a bedside vigil in which the minor fluctuations in her condition led to swings of optimism and disappointment that Darwin transmitted to Emma through daily letters. He was joined by Emma's sister-in-law Fanny (Frances Mackintosh Wedgwood), who assisted in the nursing duties, but all to no avail. Annie died on 23 April, leaving her father devastated, robbed of his favourite child – 'the joy of the household'.

Darwin left Malvern immediately, so distressed that he left the funeral and burial arrangements to Fanny.[25] Thereafter the town was inextricably linked to Annie's death. He could not return there, such was his sense of loss and the fear that the 'old thoughts would revive so vividly'.[26] Thus, when Darwin's health deteriorated in 1856, he had to look elsewhere for the water cure, and considered a visit to the Moor Park Hydropathic Establishment in Surrey[27], 'for I have great faith in treatment & no faith whatever in ordinary Doctoring'.[22] In December 1856, Emma gave birth to her tenth and last child, Charles Waring, a sickly child who never talked or walked and died of scarlet fever aged one and a half.

In April 1857, Darwin complained that 'his health had been very poor of late, & I am going in a week's time for a fortnight of hydropathy and rest. – My everlasting species-Book quite overwhelms me with work – It is beyond my powers, but I hope to live to finish it'.[28] A few days later, Darwin paid the first of several short visits to Moor Park where he gained great benefit

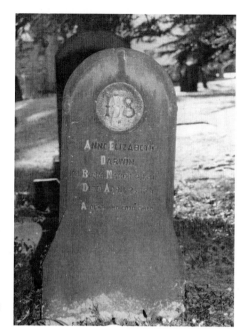

Headstone marking the grave of Anne Elizabeth Darwin. In March 1851, Darwin returned to Malvern with his terminally ill daughter, Annie. Darwin's faith in Dr Gully and the hope of a cure proved futile. Annie died on 23 April, aged ten. Darwin was devastated and could not bear the prospect of a return to Malvern, even though his confidence in the water cure remained unshaken.

from the ministrations of Dr Edward Lane, only for the vomiting to return when he got back to his research and writing at Down. Forced into company on his visits to Moor Park, Darwin displayed his sociable side, and enjoyed the conviviality of Edward and Mrs Lane, and Dr Lane's mother-in-law, Lady Elizabeth Drysdale, a well-read and elegant woman who presided over the social side of the establishment. He described the triumvirate at Moor Park as 'some of the nicest people, I have ever met'.[29] It was Lady Drysdale, no doubt, who arranged the seating plan that brought Darwin into contact with the engaging Misses Craik and Butler. They, it could be argued, represented those frequenters of hydropathic establishments much derided by Florence Nightingale. In a biting criticism, Miss Nightingale summed up hydropathy as 'a highly popular amusement amongst athletic individuals who have felt the *tedium vitae*, and those indefinite diseases which a large income and unbounded leisure are so well calculated to produce'.[30]

During 1858, Dr Lane was cited as co-respondent in a divorce suit brought by the husband of one of his patients, a Mrs Robinson, who kept a diary of her supposed adultery with Lane during a visit in 1854.[31] Although the suit was eventually abandoned, a cloud hung over Lane and Moor Park. Darwin thought Dr Lane innocent, but feared that it would ruin him.[32] He subsequently found that a much-needed visit to Moor Park in February 1859 'did not do me so much good as usual'.[33] Thus, as he wrestled with completing the *Origin*, Darwin's thoughts on future treatment were turning away from Moor Park. In March, he declared;

I am weary of my work. It is a very odd thing that I have no sensation that I overwork my brain; but facts compel me to conclude that my Brain was never formed for much thinking. – We are resolved to go for 2 or 3 months, when I have finished to Ilkley or some such place, to see if I can anyhow give my health a good start, for it certainly has been wretched of late, & has incapacitated me for everything.[34]

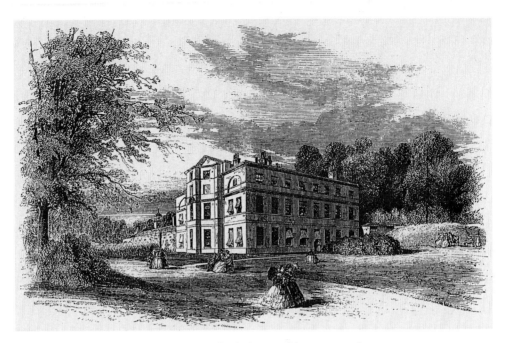

Moor Park House, Farnham, Surrey. Originally the home of the seventeenth-century statesman and essayist Sir William Temple, Moor Park was leased to Dr Edward Lane for use as a hydropathic establishment in the late 1840s. Darwin paid several visits to Moor Park, but after a course of treatment in July 1859 decided that it had not done him much good.

At the beginning of May he predicted that he would be in Ilkley in July, but then his health failed and he booked into Moor Park for an urgent course of hydropathy.[35] By July, his visit to Ilkley had not materialised, indeed he began to equivocate and asked his son William, who was on a trip to the Lake District, to investigate 'the Windermere Water-cure place; & whether any House to let close by'.[36] Apparently, Darwin was hoping to have his family accompany him on his next hydropathic excursion. Had Darwin known that the principal of the 'Windermere Hydropathic Institution' was a homeopathist and phrenologist who dabbled in mesmerism, it is unlikely that he would have pursued this particular destination.[37] Also at the beginning of July he wrote, 'I have been bad, having had two days of bad vomiting owing to the accursed Proofs – I shall have to go to Moor Park before long'.[38] Indeed, it was not long – he left home for Moor Park on 19th and returned on the 26 July.[39]

In September, Darwin received an enquiry about the family's health, to which he responded:

I cannot give a very flourishing account of Emma or of some of the children; and for myself I am in a very poor way, & quite worn out, & useless for everything. Immediately my last proof is done in 14 or 20 days; we start for 2 months' Hydropathy & rest - & perhaps that will make a man of me'.[40]

A few days later, he wrote to Mary Butler seeking her company during his treatment, explaining:

Our plans are rather undecided; but I incline strongly to go to Ilkley, but I fear, without I found it a very tempting place, that it is too late to take a house for my family; & in this case I should stop three or four weeks in the establishment, return home for a week or so, & then go to Moor Park for a few weeks, so as altogether to get a good dose of Hydropathy'.[41]

Nine days later, Darwin's mind was made up:

I start for 'Ilkley Wells Hydropathic Establishment near Otley, Yorkshire' on Oct. 3d by which time, thank God, I shall have finished last revises, index & all. My health is much broken.[42]

Notes

1   C.D. to W.D. Fox, 6 October 1859; Correspondence, 7, p. 343.

2   Lukis, J.H., *The Common Sense of the Water Cure* (Robert Hardwicke, London: 1862) pp. 104-5.

3   C.D. to J.D. Hooker, 15 October 1859; Correspondence, 7, p. 349.

4   C.D. to J.S. Henslow, 20 September 1837; Correspondence, 2, p. 47.

5   Katz-Sidlow, R.J., 'In the Darwin family tradition: another look at Charles Darwin's ill health'. *Journal of the Royal Society of Medicine*, 91: pp. 484-88.

6   See Colp Jr., R., *To be an invalid: The illness of Charles Darwin* (Chicago University Press, Chicago: 1977) p.22.

7   Colp, R.Jr., 1977, p. 101.

8   C.D. to J.D. Hooker, 5 March 1863; Correspondence, 11, p. 200.

9   C.D. to W.D. Fox, 24 October 1852; Correspondence, 5, p.100.

10   C.D. to Emma Darwin, 27 May 1848; DCP Letter 1180.

11   Barlow, N., *The Autobiography of Charles Darwin* (Collins, London: 1958) p.117.

12   C.D. to W.D. Fox, 6 February 1849; Correspondence, 4, p. 209.

13   C.D. to Richard Owen, 24 February 1849; Correspondence, 4, p. 219.

14   Gully, J.M., *The Water Cure in Chronic Disease* (Simpkin Marshall & Co. London: 1846) p.127.

15   Havins, P.J.N., *The Spas of England* (Robert Hale & Co., London: 1976).

16   The origins of the water cure are the subject of differing accounts. Some, including the Jesenik-Gräfenberg Tourist Office, favour a revelation from nature – namely, Priessnitz's observation of an injured roe deer holding its affected limb under a waterfall (see www.priessnitz. cz). Captain Claridge, an early English visitor, had a less romantic explanation. He states, 'an old man who used to practise the water cure upon animals, and occasionally upon the peasantry, was much encouraged by the elder Priessnitz; that the latter invited him to instruct his son, and that it is from this source that Vincent (Vinzenz) Priessnitz obtained his first ideas of the cold water cure'. Claridge, R.T., *Hydropathy; or the Cold Water Cure, as practised by Vincent Priessnitz, at Graefenberg, Silesia, Austria* (James Madden and Co., London: 1842) p.57.

17   Harcup, J.W., *The Malvern Water Cure* (Winsor Fox Photos, Malvern: 1992) p. 40.

18   Bostridge, M., *Florence Nightingale: The Woman And Her Legend* (Penguin Books Ltd. London: 2008) p. 77. Gully's attraction to the ladies also transcended age barriers, ultimately leading to his professional downfall. After an illicit affair with a young patient (Florence Ricardo) forty years younger than himself, he appeared as a witness at the inquest on her second husband (Charles

Bravo) who died suddenly of antimony poisoning. Gully was not incriminated but the publicity surrounding the case destroyed his practice.

19 Turner, E.S., *Taking the Cure* (Michael Joseph, London: 1967) p.165.

20 C.D. to Susan Darwin, 19 March 1849; Correspondence, 4, p.224.

21 Gully, J.M., 1846. pp. 154-162, 599.

22 C.D. to W.D. Fox, 7 July 1849; Correspondence, 4, p.246.

23 Colp Jr., R., 1977. p.44.

24 This account of Annie's final illness is taken from Litchfield, H., *Emma Darwin: A Century of Family Letters*, (John Murray, London: 1915) vol. 2, pp.132-140.

25 Annie was buried in the graveyard surrounding Malvern Priory. The headstone reads; I.H.S. (an abbreviation of Jesus) – Anne Elizabeth Darwin: Born 2 March 1841: Died April 23, 1851 – A dear and good child.

26 Moor Park House in Farnham, Surrey, is most closely associated with the seventeenth-century statesman and essayist Sir William Temple. In 1680 he bought 'Compton Hall', the name of the original property on this site, and considerably remodelled it to create Moor Park. In 1689, the author Jonathan Swift, a relative of Lady Dorothy Temple, came to Moor Park as an amanuensis to Sir William, and stayed there for ten years. See C. Hussey, 'Templum Restauratum; Sir William Temple's house and garden at Moor Park, Farnham, reconstructed'. *Country Life*, 25 November 1949.

27 C. D. to W.D. Fox, 3 October 1856; Correspondence, 6, p. 237-8.

28 C.D. to Charles Lyell, 13 April 1857; Correspondence, 6, p 377.

29 C.D. to J.D. Hooker, 25 June 1857; Correspondence, 6, p. 416.

30 Bostridge, M., 2008. p. 125.

31 *The Times*, 16 and 17 June 1858. Court Reports; Robinson v. Robinson and Lane. p.11.

32 C.D. to W.D. Fox, 24 June 1858; Correspondence, 7, p. 116.

33 Journal 1859, right. See Chronology in Correspondence, 7, p.504.

34 C.D. to W.D. Fox, 24 March 1859; Correspondence, 7, p. 268.

35 C.D. to W.E. Darwin, 5 May 1859; Correspondence, 7, p. 293; and C.D. to J.D. Hooker, 18 May 1859; Correspondence, 7, p. 299.

36 C.D. to W.E. Darwin, 7 July 1859; Correspondence, 7, p. 318.

37 The 'Windermere Hydropathic Institution' was situated at Bowness on Windermere. The Principal was Spencer Timothy Hall (1812-85), a man with dubious qualifications and suspect practices who died a pauper in Blackpool. See www.homeoint.org/morrell/british/hall.htm.

38 C.D. to J.D. Hooker, 2 July 1859; Correspondence, 7, p. 315.

39 Journal 1859, right. See Chronology in Correspondence, 7, p.505.

40 C.D. to Charles Lyell, 2 September 1859; Correspondence; 7, p. 328.

41 C.D. to Mary Butler, 11 September 1859; Correspondence, 7, p. 331.

42 C.D. to Charles Lyell, 20 September 1859; Correspondence, 7, p. 333. As it happened, Darwin left Down for Ilkley on 2nd October 1859 (Journal 1859, 38 right. See Chronology in Correspondence, 7, p. 505).

Chapter Four

The Malvern of the North

In the event, Darwin left Down House on Sunday 2 October, not arriving in Ilkley until Tuesday 4th. Given that the journey from London to Ilkley could be done in a day, he may have stayed (as he did on the return journey) with his brother Erasmus in London.[1] Leaving again on the Tuesday morning by a Great Northern train from Kings Cross to Leeds, he would have arrived at the Central Station some four and a half hours later. There he would have been met by a carriage especially dispatched from the Wells House stables.

In 1859, the only means of transport into Ilkley was by horse-drawn coach, and there were daily coaches connecting the village to Leeds and Bradford. The Leeds-Ilkley coach left from the White Horse Inn in Boar Lane, which, for anyone with luggage, meant a short cab ride from the station.[2] However, a once-a-day coach service was difficult to co-ordinate with a long train journey. Thus many visitors to Ilkley extended their train journey north of Leeds to the station at Arthington, a village only eleven miles from Ilkley, to take advantage of an easier and quicker, but not necessarily safer, coach ride along the Wharfe Valley.[3] Darwin's journey from Leeds, however, would have been even more convenient.

The journey was a picturesque one. After the steady and comparatively gentle ascent out of Airedale through Headingley to the village of Bramhope, the road took a double bend through a cutting and, quite suddenly, a magnificent panorama of the Wharfe Valley opened out below as the road led down to Otley. This road was built in 1841, and the new route provided a much shallower gradient than the old road linking Otley to Bramhope village. With such a view, Darwin could not fail to be impressed by the final leg of his journey to this *terra incognita*.

The turnpike wound its way through the bustling market town of Otley, to run alongside the River Wharfe. A few miles on, it passed through the textile manufacturing village of Burley-in-Wharfedale, before finally approaching Ilkley. As the carriage rounded the final bend in the Otley-Ilkley road, Darwin would have seen his destination, Wells House, standing prominently on the hillside above the village. Higher up the moor, in those days called Rombald's, or Rumbold Moor, stood the low white-washed old bath-house known as White Wells, still a favourite Ilkley destination, and high above that he could see the great outcrops of millstone grit that form Ilkley Crags. Fifteen minutes later, after a laboured climb up Wells Road, the carriage arrived at Wells House, where porters in their dark-green livery would have shown Darwin into the impressive entrance hall, and followed on with his luggage.

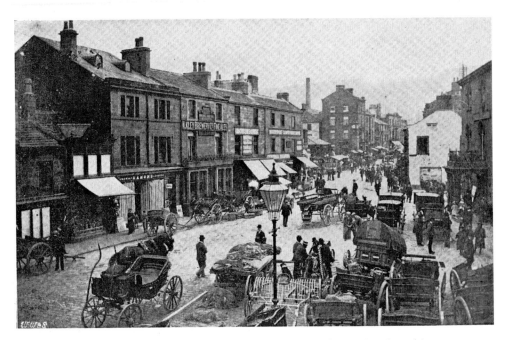

Kirkgate, Otley. Darwin would have passed through this bustling market town and coaching centre on his way from Leeds to Ilkley.

Over the next few days, Darwin familiarised himself with the facilities, the routine and the rules of the house. Besides the baths, the diet and the draughts of water, he was well aware that exercise was an integral part of the hydropathic regime. While gymnastics were on offer at the hotel, the prospect of any more than five minutes engaged in voluntary contortions or whirling dumb-bells would have filled Darwin with dread. Walking offered a far more sensible and enjoyable alternative. Although Darwin favoured a gentle stroll around the Sand Walk while at Down House, Dr Smith asserted that for a walk to be effective it must not be on the level. It was the guru, Priessnitz, who declared 'We must have hills', and hills were at the very doorstep of Wells House.[4] As an introduction to the rigours ahead, guests were encouraged to walk up the donkey track to White Wells.

The fame of Ilkley's cold water as a cure-all long preceded the nineteenth-century rise of hydropathy. White Wells was erected in the first half of the seventeenth century around a plunge bath filled with water from one of several springs that issued from Rombald's Moor.[5] At first the building was merely an enclosing wall that offered some privacy and shelter from the wind, but gave little encouragement to those potential bathers who were wavering over the whole idea of immersion in cold water. The water was certainly cold. It was piped from an underground source into the bath, and the temperature varied little, being around 40°F (4°C) both winter and summer. The coldness of the water rendered it particularly effective. Writing in 1709, a Dr Richardson of Bierley Hall, Bradford, was disparaging about Ilkley as a place but complimentary about the bath: 'Ilkley now is a very mean place, and is equally dirty and insignificant, and chiefly famous for a cold well, which has done very remarkable cures in scrofulous cases by bathing, and in drinking of it'.[6]

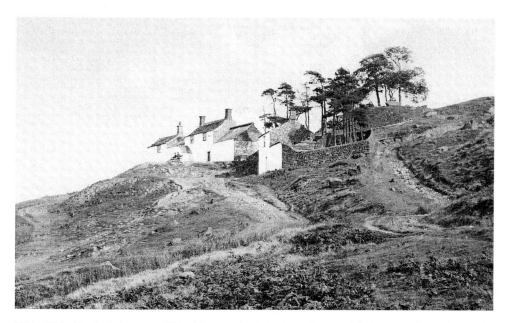

White Wells. The bath-house on Ilkley Moor was built in the early seventeenth century but considerably enlarged and enhanced in the eighteenth. Its reputation for cold-water cures gave a Leeds businessman, Hamer Stansfeld, the idea that hydropathy could flourish in Ilkley.

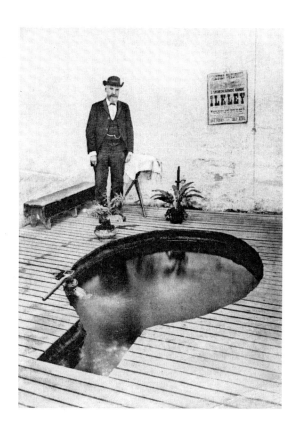

The plunge-bath at White Wells. It held 1,150 gallons of water that issued from an underground spring. The water was ideal for cold immersion, being around 4°C in both summer and winter.

In the eighteenth century, the original plunge bath was rebuilt and the buildings were extended to enclose a second bath (to offer separate baths for men and women), dressing rooms and living accommodation.[7] At this time, the larger of the two baths had an inscription over it: 'This holds 1,150 gallons, and fills in 13 minutes'.[8] When taking a bath, the usual practice was to undergo immersion for up to ten minutes, but, 'the shock on plunging into Ilkley bath is excessive, and an irresistible impulse to escape from its influence is the first sensation produced'.[9] Eventual escape from the bath was followed by brisk towelling by the bath-attendant. This vigorous activity, and the subsequent reunion with his or her clothes, induced the anticipated 'reaction' in the bather. The sense of well-being this engendered, coupled no doubt with relief at surviving the cold-water 'shock', had a distinctly therapeutic effect, even if this was no more than a particularly powerful placebo response.

In 1775, Thomas Jeffrey's map of Yorkshire marked the site of White Wells as a 'spaw', a dialect version of the generic term 'spa'. This is a misnomer because – as discussed in the last chapter – the water issuing from the drinking fountain behind the bath-house contained no dissolved minerals. It could not therefore, in any conventional sense, be claimed to have 'medicinal qualities' and so strictly speaking did not qualify as a spa.[10] Nevertheless its purity became its overriding virtue. Writing in 1830, Dr Thomas Shaw, a member of the Royal College of Surgeons, admitted that the water, 'has frequently been analysed; but the decomposition always proved that it contains no medicinal quality'. But Shaw turned the apparent deficiency into an advantage: 'In my opinion, it is its purity and softness only which makes it more efficacious, by passing sooner to the utmost and finest limits of the circulation, than any water known'.[11] Ilkley water was therefore ideal for hydrotherapy, a notion not lost on an itinerant medical man, Dr Granville, when he visited the village during his tour of the Northern Spas some time before 1841:

Here, then, is a proper field and an opportune appliance for establishing in this county a branch of that system of cold water cure, or Hydrosudomania, which has of late years become a universal topic of conversation, and a subject of the most marvellous stories in Germany: I allude to the practice of the Silesian peasant, Vincent Priessnitz, who has founded, on the rugged side of the hill in Graefenberg, in Bohemia – a spot nearly resembling this of Ilkley – a new Hygeian temple, wherein all diseases are said to be cured by the internal and the external use of cold water, issuing from the recesses of this native mountain.[12]

Granville's remarkably perceptive assessment was to become a reality just a few years later.

On reaching White Wells in 1859, there was no special incentive for the Wells House guests to drink the water. After all, they had the identical water *gratis* and *ad libitum* down at the hotel. Likewise there would have been no need for them to take a bath amid these rustic amenities when they had spent the morning having treatment in the luxury of their own temple to Hygeia in Wells House.[13] They would, however, no doubt have availed themselves of the bench seats outside the bath-house (both to admire the view and to catch their breath again after the steady slog up the donkey track).

At a height of 690ft above sea level and 460ft above the River Wharfe, the view was a rewarding one. Ilkley itself occupied only a small part of the panorama. Its 1,000 or so inhabitants occupied just 190 houses clustered around the main axes of the Otley-Skipton turnpike and

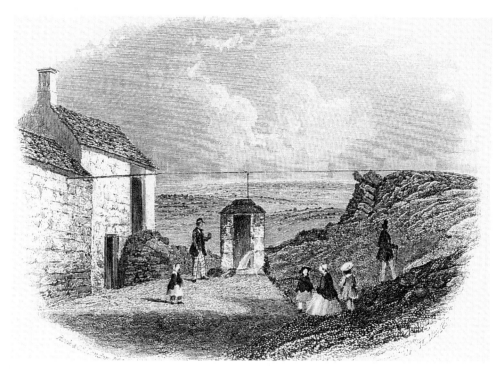

The drinking fountain behind White Wells, May 1857. The water contained 'no medicinal quality' but because of its purity passed more readily into 'the finest limits of the circulation than any water known'. Thus, Ilkley water reached the parts that other waters could not reach!

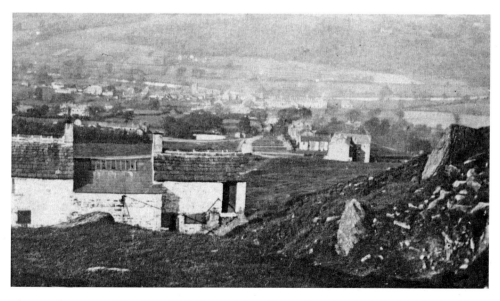

The view from above White Wells. Wells Terrace (where Darwin lodged with his family) is in the right foreground while just above the central part of the bath-house, Wells House Stables can be seen with the upper mill dam to its right (east). (Gordon Burton)

Brook Street, running at right angles to it. On the far side of the river, Myddleton Lodge stood in splendid isolation above the woods. The village was merely incidental to the vista presented by mid-Wharfedale, from the sweep of hills behind Addingham in the west, to the higher hills flanking the valley beyond Bolton Abbey and Burnsall, around to Beamsley Beacon and the expanse of moor behind Langbar and Middleton, and onwards behind Askwith and Denton as the valley broadened out. Denton Hall, ancient home of the Fairfax family, could be seen in the distance on the southern flank of the valley. The estate was sold to the Ibbetsons in 1716, and in 1845 the hall passed to the Wyvill family. In 1859 it was the home of Marmaduke Wyvill, Member of Parliament for the Richmond (Yorkshire) constituency and a leading chess master.[14] In the far distance, the distinctive outline of Almscliff Crag interrupted the sky-line. The view to the east was curtailed by the flank of the moor running up to the Hangingstone quarries. Although Ben Rhydding Hydro was less than a mile away, it was hidden behind this slope of land, as were the great Cow and Calf Rocks – the iconic rock formation that served to symbolise Ilkley for generations of walkers and climbers, and does so to the present day.

There was little in the Ilkley of 1859 to engage the attention of visitors, a positive advantage for the discipline of Wells House. It was reported that in Ilkley, 'late dinners, balls, concerts, and such like dissipations, are unknown… In the establishment, a glass of wine, except as medicine, is inadmissible; and harmless pic-nics, mild charades, and innocent quadrilles, are the most daring excitements'.[15] Nevertheless, for many of the guests, purchasing stamps at the Post Office was a popular errand, and a good reason to stroll into the village.

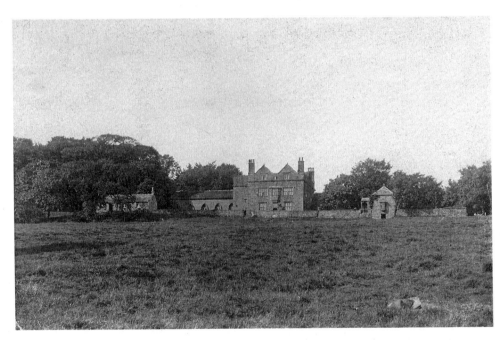

Myddelton Lodge. The Middeltons, Lords of the Manor of Ilkley, succeeded to the Stockeld estate between Spofforth and Wetherby in 1318 and this became their principal residence. When staying in Ilkley, the Middeltons initially lived in Low Hall but transferred to their Elizabethan hunting lodge, Myddelton Hall, in the late sixteenth century. (Gordon Burton)

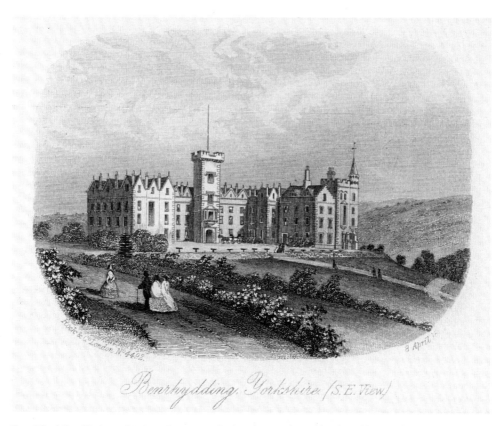

Benrhydding, Yorkshire (S.E. View)

Ben Rhydding Hydropathic Hotel. In 1859, the hotel was enlarged by the addition of a north wing, seen on the right with the small spire. At the same time, Dr Macleod signalled his departure from the strict cold-water regime by building a separate block containing Turkish baths.

The guests took a tree-lined path that ran from the hotel alongside the lower drive down to the stables and the two cottages that flanked the entrance to the stable-yard. Skirting around the top-side of the pond that formed the upper mill-dam, the path joined Wells Road some distance from the top, with the houses of West View ahead.[16] The lowest of these, indistinguishable from the others apart from a sign, was a beer-house run by William Beanlands. On the west side (left of the descending walker) were two corn mills, the lower having a separate and smaller dam, and nearby a white-washed thatched house occupied by the Downs family, like many houses in the village offering board and lodging of a modest sort. Shortly thereafter on the right, a drive ran up to the vicarage – Skelda Grange, built in 1848. The original vicarage opposite the church had been declared unfit for the vicar, the Reverend John Snowdon, but remained in use for many years afterwards as accommodation for the schoolmaster! Opposite the entrance to Skelda Grange stood a small thatched cottage owned by Sarah Batty, where the vicar and his family lodged while the new vicarage was under construction. Behind this cottage, the mill stream continued in a deep rock-strewn gully – Mill Ghyll – and then disappeared into a culvert (built in 1854) that took it beneath Brook Street to emerge beyond the turnpike road in another gully that ran down to the Wharfe.

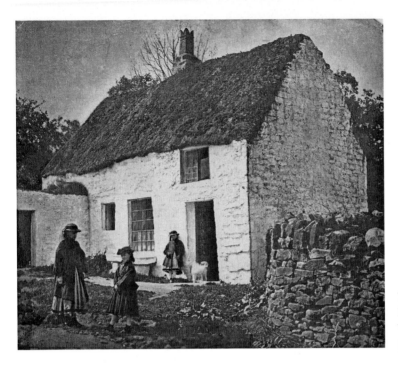

Thomas and Emma
Downs' cottage,
Wells Road.
(Gordon Burton)

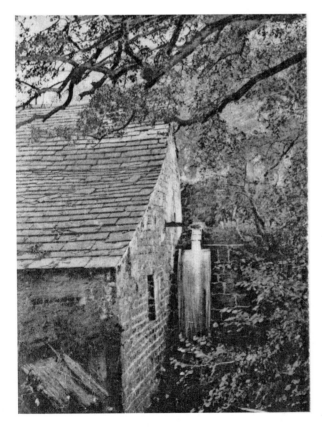

The lower corn mill in Mill Ghyll.

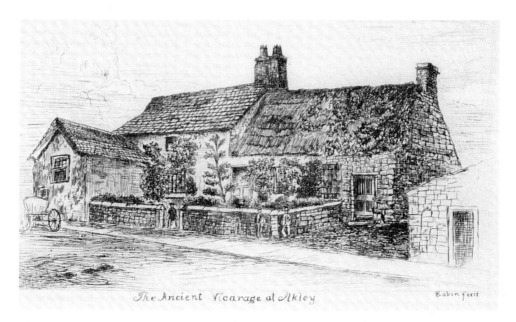

The Ancient Vicarage at Ilkley   Robin fecit

The 'ancient vicarage at Ilkley'. So ancient and ruinous that when a new vicar was appointed in 1842, he declared it unfit for habitation and rented a house until a new vicarage had been built.

Towards the foot of Wells Road, a short row of five houses stood on the eastern side. The bottom house was demolished to create a site for the York City and County Bank (now the HSBC), built in 1905, but the other houses still survive – albeit as shops. The route to the Post Office lay ahead down Brook Street. To the right, the then anonymous road that was to become Station Road in 1865, contained on its south side a row of dilapidated cottages, soon to be pulled down to make way for the Midland and North View Hotels. The latter was re-named 'The Station' following the construction of the railway extension to Skipton and the demise of the original Station Hotel in Brook Street. A short distance farther on stood a substantial farmhouse, Sedbergh Farm, which together with its outbuildings was demolished in the 1890s to provide land for Ilkley's municipal buildings. Back at the top of Brook Street, the narrow lane running west – Green Lane, now The Grove – contained only two houses: Hartley's farmhouse, and another old thatch that was reputedly Ilkley's first Post Office (before the era of the 'penny-post') and an occasional holiday retreat for the illustrious Madame Tussaud.[17]

Entering Brook Street, the visitor would have been struck by its breadth, little thinking that the building lines were established when the street had a brook running down its middle. A row of houses occupied the lower half of the east side of the street, with just one converted into a shop. These houses are largely intact today, although their lower parts are heavily disguised by shop fascias and signs. At the foot of the street, the building of the Crescent Hotel was well-advanced and it opened for business in 1860. The west side was an untidy mix of older buildings, including a cruck-built cottage converted into a shop and Hawksworth's old ivy-clad barn, but towards the bottom was a new addition to the street scene – Brook Terrace, a handsome block of four shops with two floors for housing above, erected in 1855.

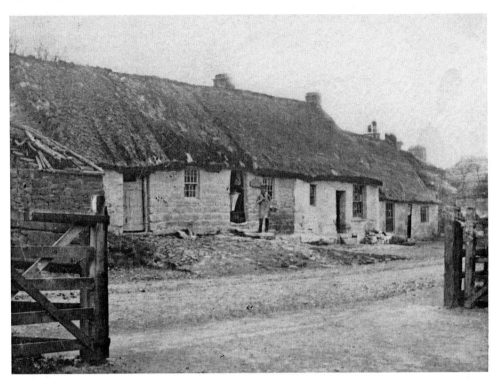

Old cottages on what is now Station Road, where the Midland Hotel stands. (Gordon Burton)

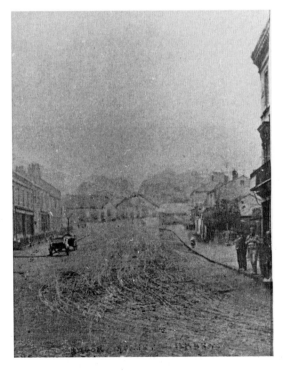

Brook Street, looking south. The stream that originally ran down the middle of the street was culverted in 1855. A few of the houses on the east side have been converted into shops, but the west side remains a ramshackle affair apart from Brook Terrace, the short parade of shops just entering the right of the photograph. (Gordon Burton)

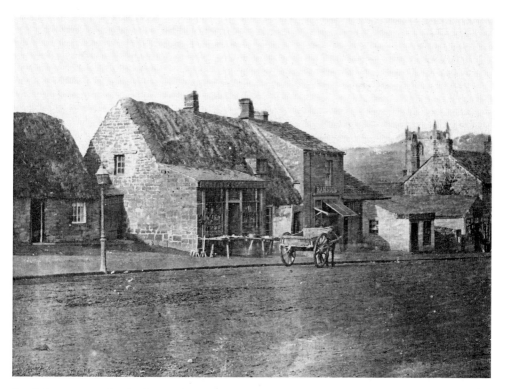

Brook Street, west side. The shop in the centre belonged to George Ickringill, a grocer. The shop was converted from a small cruck-built cottage of considerable antiquity. (Gordon Burton)

On the turnpike road opposite the foot of Brook Street stood two public houses, the Star Inn and the Wheatsheaf, separated by a narrow entry. Behind the Star Inn was the original gas-works; it was a small affair, founded by the Ilkley Gas Lighting Company in 1856, but its tall chimney became something of a local landmark. The Otley Road (now Leeds Road) contained a smithy, then managed by Christopher Cocker, but indelibly linked to the name of Robert Collyer, an Ilkley blacksmith who emigrated to America in 1850 and who, in February 1859, became a Unitarian minister in Chicago. Collyer was to become a major pulpit figure in the United States and ranks as one of Ilkley's 'favourite sons'. The Otley Road was lined by a scattering of houses and workshops ending with Holly Bank House, a lodging house and home to the Dobson family. John Dobson was a friend and mentor of Robert Collyer and with his brother, Francis, ran a coach service into Leeds and Bradford. Earlier in 1859, their elder brother, Michael Dobson, had erected the Craiglands Hydropathic Hotel on land off Cowpasture Road.[18] This modest hydropathic establishment was the first of a wave of smaller hydros built between 1860 and the 1880s (namely the Troutbeck, The Spa, Rockwood House, Marlborough House, and the Stoney Lea) that catered for the middle classes. Lower down Cowpasture Road, clusters of houses in Mount Pleasant and Belle Vue were almost all given over to lodging and boarding houses.

Turning left from Brook Street into the turnpike (at this point known as Kirkgate, nowadays Church Street), the visitor was confronted by the ancient parish church, surrounded by its

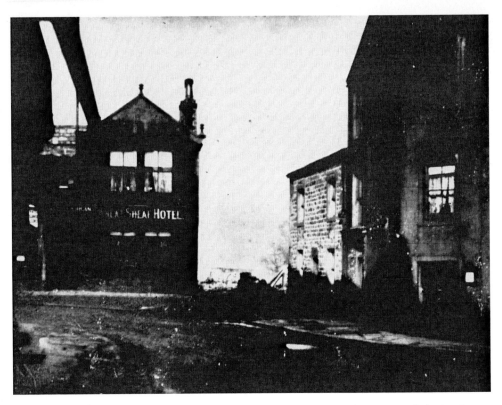

The Wheatsheaf Hotel at the top of Kirkgate (Church Street). On the right is the side of The Star Inn. The turnpike road from Otley undertook a dog-leg around the Star to enter Kirkgate.

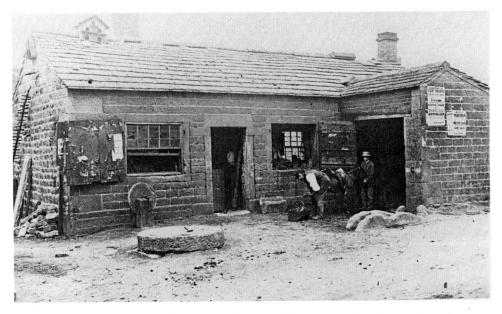

The smithy in Otley Road at which Robert Collyer served his apprenticeship. (Gordon Burton)

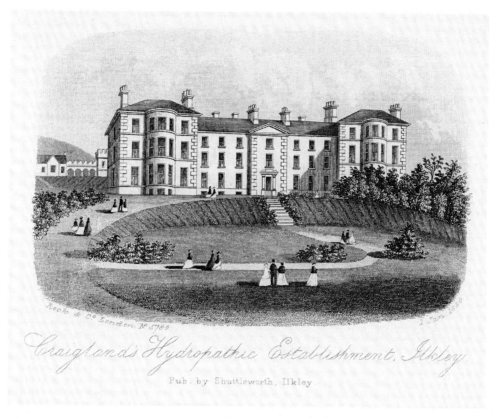

Craiglands Hydropathic Establishment, Ilkley.

Pub. by Shuttleworth, Ilkley

The Craiglands Hydropathic Hotel opened in 1859. It was erected by Michael Dobson, from Holly Bank House, Otley Road, and partly financed by Dr Macleod of Ben Rhydding.

dismal graveyard. The squat fifteenth-century tower was the oldest intact part of the structure, but three Saxon crosses standing sentinel near the entrance bore testimony to its early origins. The entrance porch enclosed a much-modified Norman arch, while a stone effigy of the fourteenth-century Peter de Middelton lay in repose in a side chapel. The church, dedicated to All Saints, was furnished with box-pews of great antiquity and in a state of disrepair, and the only source of heat was a single stove in the centre of the nave that did nothing to encourage attendance during the winter months. The general air of dilapidation that characterised the church in 1859 was to change over the next two years, for in 1860-1861 it was virtually reconstructed.

Kirkgate was lined by shops which on the north side were converted from old houses and cottages, one bearing the date 1709 over its doorway. Through an archway lay Castle Yard containing the old 'Castle' (nowadays inappropriately called the Manor House), a yeoman farmer's house of fourteenth-century origin but largely rebuilt in the seventeenth. By the mid-nineteenth century, the once grand house was sub-divided into five diminutive dwellings. These and the remaining cottages in Castle Yard contained an ill-assortment of rough-tongued wool-combers, layabouts and ragamuffins, and were definitely off-limits for the genteel visitor. The succession of shops on the south side of Kirkgate was interrupted by two old buildings, the Rose & Crown Inn – the terminus for the coaches from Leeds – and

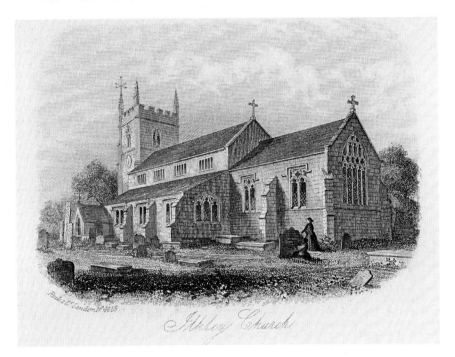

Itchley Church

All Saints Parish Church. The church was in a dilapidated condition in 1859 but underwent major reconstruction over ten months in 1860-61. The nave was lengthened by 16ft, and the whole of the south aisle and main entrance porch demolished and rebuilt.

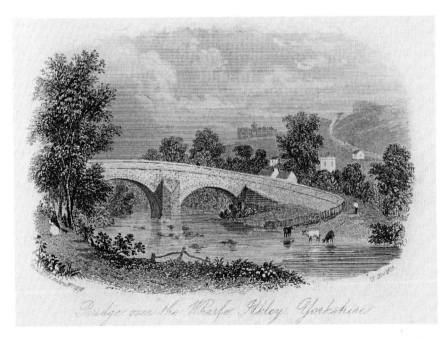

Bridge over the Wharfe Ilkley Yorkshire

The Old Bridge, viewed from up-river, 1855. In this rather fanciful depiction, Ben Rhydding Hydro dominates the distant skyline.

the ancient vicarage. The vicarage porch had at one time served as a 'dispensary', known by the locals as 't'old Charity Hole', where Curate Fenton doled out simple remedies in the 1830s. At the bottom of the street stood John Seanor's dairy and farmhouse, an elegant Queen Anne building called Box Tree Cottage (*c.* 1710). Opposite, Bridge Lane ran down to the old bridge (dating from 1675), at that time the only crossing point over the Wharfe, and giving access to the Middelton estate and the hamlets of Nessfield and Langbar. It was from an old thatch and the adjacent 'stable' in Bridge Lane that William Rigg ran the string of donkeys that trudged up to White Wells. The lane also contained a much more substantial property, Castle House, a handsome three-storey building of around 1740.

After Bridge Lane, the turnpike became Addingham Road, and on the opposite corner stood the Lister's Arms Hotel – called the 'New Inn' for some years after its opening in 1825, but no longer new in 1859. Dr Granville, the peripatetic commentator on the spas of England, was complimentary:

The New Inn is, for so retired a place as Ilkley, very respectable. There is a large public room in it, and the back looks towards the rich and smiling ascent leading to the moor. In front, the road is a great posting thoroughfare from the West to the East Riding – from Skipton, or even the Lakes, to

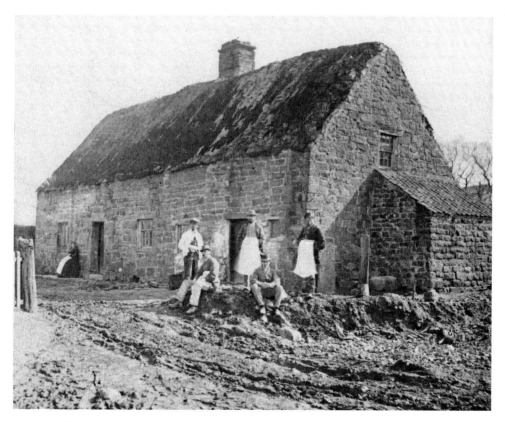

Hartley's old farm house, then referred to (wrongly) as 'The Manor House' was the only building on the south side of Green Lane (The Grove) in 1859. (Gordon Burton)

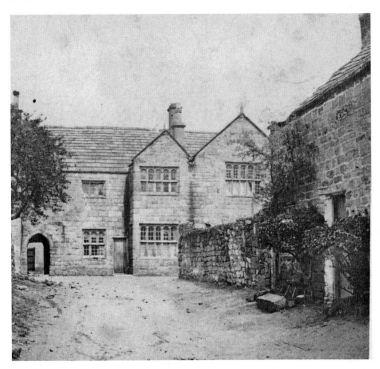

'The Castle' – a former yeoman farmer's house that by 1859 had been divided into small tenements. The building is now the Manor House Museum and Art Gallery.
(Gordon Burton)

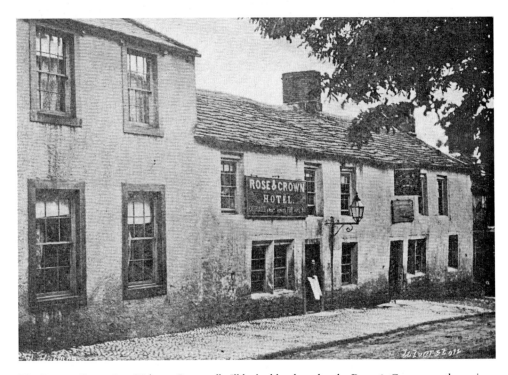

The Rose & Crown Inn, Kirkgate. Reputedly Ilkley's oldest hostelry, the Rose & Crown was the major coaching inn in 1859. The landlord at that time was Mr William Kendall.

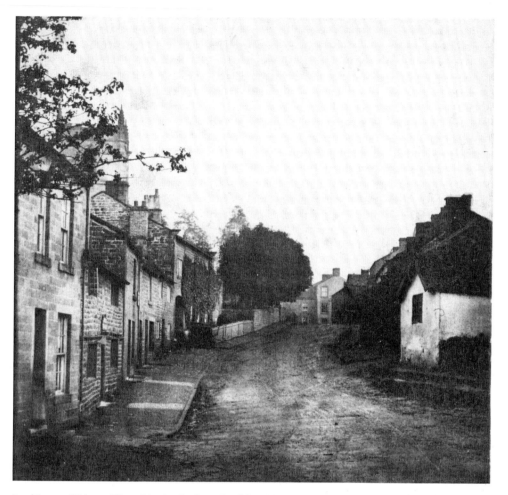

Looking up Kirkgate. The white-washed porch of the old vicarage is seen on the right. In the 1830s, this had been used as a dispensary by the curate George Fenton, and was known by the locals as 't'old Charity Hole'. (Gordon Burton)

Leeds and York. As many as thirty dine in this room at a table d'hôte, in the summer, when some of the most renowned trout are served up, fresh caught in the Wharfe, such as scarcely any other river in the north is said to rival; game, also, as may be supposed, is plentiful; and during grouse-shooting no moor can offer a richer treat than Rumbold side and topping.[19]

Farther down Addingham Road, on the other side, stood the old Grammar School, built around 1635 and still giving rudimentary instruction in the three 'R's' to those boys and girls whose parents could afford the penny per week. Beyond the school was the White House, home of the Post Office. The post-master was Richard Vickers and he, with help from his four sisters, had run the business since 1838. Self-evidently, the postal service was of considerable interest to Darwin. At the time, Ilkley was a sub-office of Otley. The letters, 'from all parts', were received in Otley from Arthington station at 7.15 a.m., and a mailcart left Otley for Burley, Ben Rhydding and Ilkley at 7.50 a.m. Letters posted in London arrived in Ilkley the following day, and vice versa.[20] The mail would be delivered to Wells House by 10 a.m. The mail carrier, George Hickman, had to remain in Ilkley all day to await the return journey to Otley at 5.00 p.m. He was put up, with his trap, at the Listers Arms Hotel, no doubt enjoying ample refreshment in the meantime.[21] Outgoing mail taken down to the Ilkley Office would be received in Otley by 6.00 p.m, sorted and dispatched to Arthington at 7.15 p.m.

The attraction of the Post Office for visitors to Wells House had little to do with posting letters. The explanation lay with the Misses Vickers for they, in addition to their occasional duties with the Royal Mail, were pastry-cooks and confectioners – indeed, the Post Office was in a corner of a confectionary shop. A sugar-deprived visitor at Wells House explained:

> Entrance is unnecessary for the mere posting of a letter, but stamps can only be obtained from behind the counter. The consequences of this proximity to danger may be supposed. Although letter writing is discouraged by the doctor, and in some cases actually forbidden, it is astonishing what a number of people are continually in want of stamps. The Post-office is, in fact, a regular trap for water-patients, baited with Queen's heads; and so successful is it in its action that purchasing stamps has become a recognized euphemism for investing in toffee.[22]

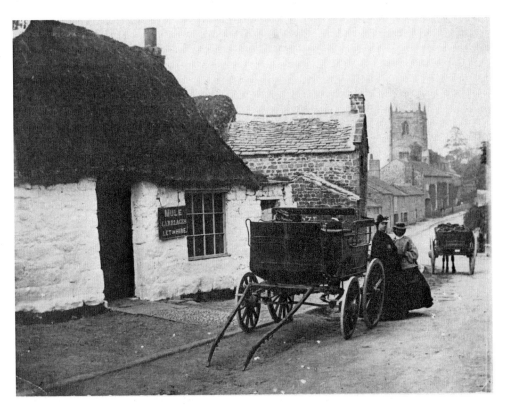

Old thatch where carriages could be hired, and next door an old stone cottage, in Addingham Road opposite the Lister's Arms Hotel. (Gordon Burton)

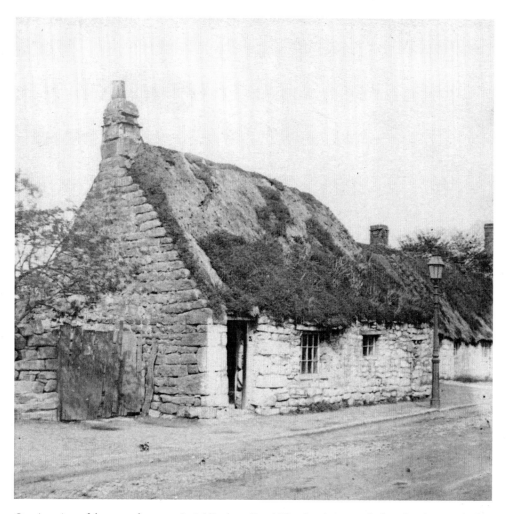

Continuation of the row of cottages in Addingham Road. The thatch was made from heather in which self-planted house leeks and saxifrage flourished in the spring. The floors were either flagged or made of compacted earth; there was no water supply or sanitation. (Gordon Burton)

Suitably sweetened, the visitor would usually return whence they came by foot or take a carriage, or even a donkey, back up the hill. The enthusiastic walker, particularly those of a non-conformist persuasion, would no doubt extend their stroll farther along Addingham Road to see the Wesleyan Chapel. The chapel was at the corner of Chapel Lane (now Bolton Bridge Road) and still stands, the gable end of the building clearly visible above the car showroom below. The chapel was erected in 1834 and had a characteristic simple and austere design – an undistinguished building lacking a single redeeming architectural feature. Inside, it was packed with undecorated pitch-pine pews and had a balcony running around three sides, the building holding up to 300 worshippers. By 1859, the Wesleyans were ill at ease with their homely, inelegant chapel and were looking for a new site on which to build something more distinguished. A suitable piece of land became available in the first Middelton land sale of 1867, and they erected a much more imposing Victorian Gothic pile in

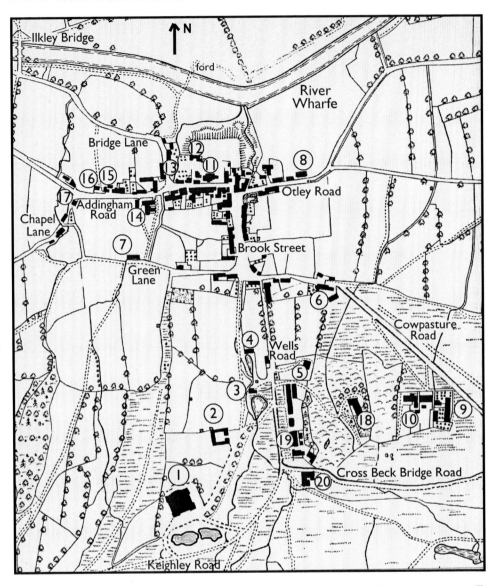

Ilkley in 1859: 1. Wells House Hydropathic Establishment; 2. Wells House stables; 3. Upper corn mill; 4. Lower corn mill; 5. The new Vicarage (Skelda Grange); 6. Sedbergh Farm; 7. Green Lane Cottage; 8. Holly Bank House; 9. Mount Pleasant; 10. Belle Vue; 11. All Saints Church; 12. 'The Castle' (Manor House); 13. The Donkey House and Castle House; 14. The Lister's Arms Hotel; 15. The old Grammar School; 16. The White House (Post Office); 17. Wesleyan Chapel; 18. Dixon's Hall; 19. 'The Crescent' (Usher's boarding house); 20. Wells Terrace. (Based on the Heritage Cartography map of Ilkley, 1847)

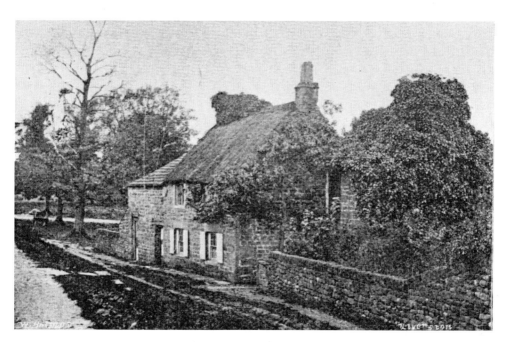

The other notable building in Green Lane, this one on the north side, was Green Lane Cottage. This was Ilkley's first Post Office before it moved to the White House in Addingham (Skipton) Road, its location in 1859.

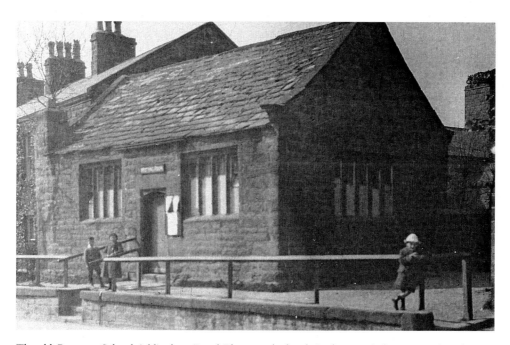

The old Grammar School, Addingham Road. Photographed early in the twentieth century, when the building was used as a meeting hall by the Christian Brethren. It closed as a school in 1872. In 1859 it was flanked by thatched cottages, that on its western side being the White House, the site of the Post Office.

Wells Road. Turning left at the chapel, the walker entered Chapel Lane but did not continue to the row of mean and dilapidated cottages along the lane, but took the footpath ahead to join up with the end of Green Lane, and return to Wells Road.

Once in Wells Road, the visitor returning to Wells House might opt for the more gradual climb to the top of the road with the intention of entering the hotel by the main drive off Keighley Road (as the continuation of Wells Road was called). In doing so, the vacant building plots on either side of West View House would give glimpses of Dixon's Hall, a Regency villa in extensive grounds to the east.[23] The next house was called 'The Crescent' – a large boarding house run by John Usher and his sister Elizabeth. The house, built in 1833-34, was first occupied by their father, Edward Usher, and it was in his time that the 'The Crescent' provided accommodation for Ilkley's first hydropathic doctor.[24]

When the Leeds businessman Hamer Stansfeld returned from Gräfenberg, filled with the joys of cold-water treatment, he decided to establish the water cure somewhere in the environs of Leeds. Given the reputation of Ilkley as a minor 'spa', his choice was a predictable one. Stansfeld installed the Austrian physician Rischanek, hired to set up a hydropathic practice in Ilkley, in Usher's boarding house in April 1843.[25] Dr Rischanek used the baths at White Wells for his patients, but these had to be paid for, and Edward Usher and the other boarding-house keepers took their profits on the patient's accommodation. It soon dawned on Stansfeld that a special 'hydropathic

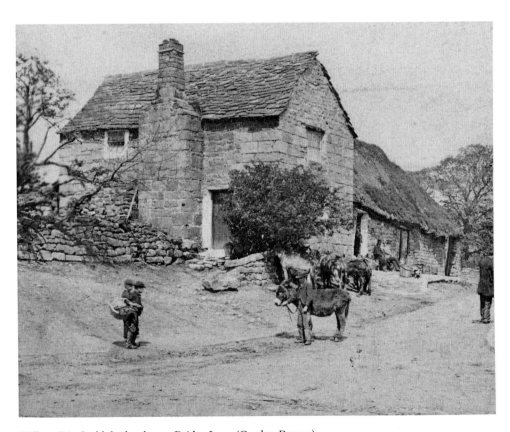

William Rigg's old donkey house, Bridge Lane. (Gordon Burton)

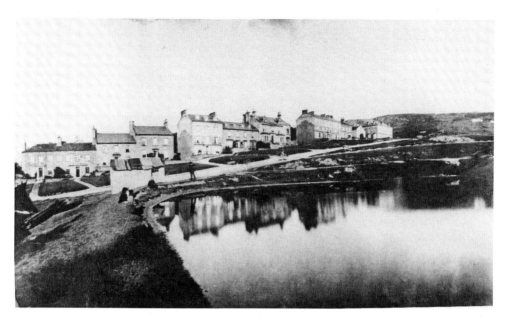

The houses of West View, Wells Road, seen across part of the upper mill dam. (Roland Wade)

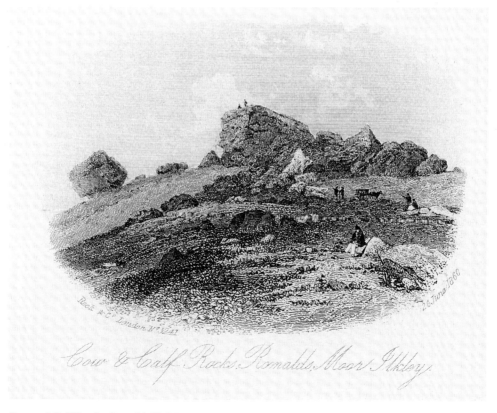

Cow and Calf Rocks, Rom(b)alds Moor.

hotel', equipped with its own baths, would be a more profitable enterprise.[26] In conjunction with four other Leeds businessmen, Stansfeld purchased land above the then hamlet of Wheatley, and erected the Ben Rhydding Hydropathic Establishment (which opened in May 1844).

Above Usher's was another boarding-house, Moor Lodge, built in 1829 and owned by Elizabeth Beanlands. Next door was a white-washed eighteenth-century house, Moor Cottage. Built around 1727 and occupied by Elizabeth's sister, Sarah, this was also a lodging-house. Moor Cottage adjoined the first house opening onto Cross Beck Bridge Road (now Crossbeck Road), a cottage that became No. 1 South View. Separated by a vacant plot, the next house was Laburnum Cottage, built in 1827, which became No. 5 South View.[27] Across the road from South View was Wells Terrace (now called 'Hillside Court'), which in 1859 was a recently-completed building that comprised three houses belonging to a Mr Marshall Hainsworth. Two of the houses faced west, and one faced north. The latter house was to become the temporary residence of Charles Darwin and his family.

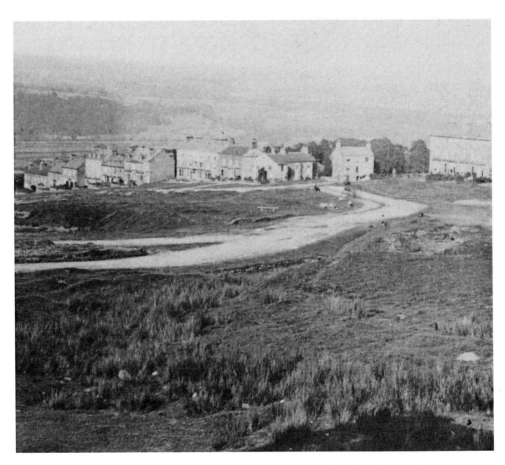

West View, Wells Road, seen from the Keighley Road near Wells House. On the right is Wells Terrace. Across Cross Beck Bridge Road, the vacant plot between Moor Cottage and Laburnum Cottage is clearly seen. Down Wells Road, the next house is Moor Lodge, followed by Usher's boarding house – 'The Crescent' (now Rombald's Hotel). (Gordon Burton)

Notes

1   Journal 1859. See Chronology in Correspondence, 7, p.505.

2   *The Ilkley Visitor and Wharfedale Advertiser*, Issue 2, June 1854. p. 1.

3   While providing the easiest route, the Arthington-Ilkley omnibus service was the subject of considerable public disquiet. On 26 September 1859, an overloaded coach from Ilkley crashed near Arthington causing serious injury to a lady passenger. A newspaper report stated that, 'The omnibus is frequently crowded to excess, and the passengers placed in imminent danger through the recklessness of those who have charge of the rotten vehicles employed to work'. *Leeds Mercury*, 1 October 1859, Supplement, p.1.

4   Lukis, J.H., *The Common Sense of the Water Cure: A popular description of Life & Treatment in a Hydropathic Establishment* (Robert Hardwicke, London: 1862) p.129.

5   The date of construction of White Wells is not recorded. There is mention of 'the Wells' in the Addingham Parish Council Records of 1656 and this is considered to be a reference to the 'White Wells' at Ilkley. In the records of the Overseer of the Poor (Joshua Dawson) his receipts and disbursements for 1655 state, 'To Richard Shires towards his charge of carrying his daughter a catiffe (caitiff – a miserable or wretched person) to the Wells for recovery of her health – 2 shillings' (Addingham St. Peter Parish Records 1612-1977, West Yorkshire Archive Service, Bradford).

6   Richardson's letter was published in Hearne's edition of Leland's *Itinerary* (Oxford, 1710). See Collyer, R., and Turner, J.H., *Ilkley: Ancient and Modern* (William Walker & Sons, Otley: 1885) p. 245.

7   An account book drawn up by a Mr. Smith of Addingham covering the period 1738-48 details the expenses incurred in maintaining an orphaned nephew, Steven Smith, at Ilkley Well while he had bath treatment. In 1741 he spent the following on Steven's behalf: '9 weeks Table at Ilkley Well – 12s., For Attendance There and Washing – 13s 6d., To the Well Man for Bathing – 4s 6d., Pocket money and Expenses at Ilkley – 2s. 6d'. This indicates that the tenants at the Well also took in boarders. DD61: Smith of Addingham (Box 60,61 BRA692), Yorkshire Archaeological Society archives.

8   Collyer, R., and Turner, J.H., 1885. p. 245.

9   Granville, A.B., *The Spas of England, and Principal Sea-Bathing Places: Northern Spas* (Henry Colburn, London: 1841) p. 388.

10 Subsequent analyses have revealed several dissolved minerals in the water. For instance, an analysis carried out in 1914 revealed iron (0.16 parts per million), calcium (16.95 p.p.m.), magnesium (9.01 p.p.m.) and sodium (11.9 p.p.m.) among other dissolved constituents. See Department of Scientific and Industrial Research: *Geology of the country between Bradford and Skipton*, H.M.S.O., 1953. p. 149.

11 Shaw, T., *A history of Wharfdale* (sic). (William Walker, Otley: 1830) p. 75.

12 Granville, A.B., 1841. p. 390.

13 This runs contrary to the description by Desmond and Moore of Darwin's hydropathic treatment in Ilkley: 'The baths were at the spring, in a stubby brick terrace (?) on a nearby hill dappled with deciduous trees. Donkeys bore the invalids there from the mansion (Wells House), a twenty-minute ride'. (Desmond, A., and Moore, J., *Darwin*, Michael Joseph, London, 1991; p. 476). The only logical reason for invalids staying at Wells House to go up to White Wells was to admire the view. Around 1856, the directors of Wells House also took a lease on White Wells and thereafter administered and received the proceeds for the baths. During his tenure as physician, Dr Smith was paid by the Ilkley Bath Charity for the baths taken at White Wells by Charity patients. In 1862, this

amounted to £25 4s 2d. Interestingly, Mr B.B. Popplewell, chairman of the Wells House directors, was the signatory to the Ilkley Charity accounts. *Leeds Mercury*, 17 April 1862. p. 1.

14 Speight, H., *Upper Wharfedale*. (Elliot Stock, London: 1900) p. 181.

15 Lukis, J.H., 1862. p. 85.

16 West View was known as Dixon's Terrace at this time. The description of Ilkley in 1859 that follows is based on the 1:4500 O.S. First series, Yorkshire: Sheet 169 – surveyed 1847, and the 1857 Post Office Directory of the West Riding of Yorkshire, part 1. pp 330-31; taking into account the 1861 census returns and the Middelton Land Sale map of April 1867, prepared by Smith and Gotthardt, Land Agents and Surveyors, Bradford.

17 Speight, H., 1900. p. 218.

18 The name 'Craiglands' is an allusion to Ilkley Crags. The word 'craig', meaning a rocky cliff or outcrop, was a largely Scottish usage. Interestingly, Darwin uses the name 'Salisbury Craigs' when he describes the famous Edinburgh geological feature (*Life and Letters*, I, p. 41).

19 Granville, A.B., 1841. p. 384.

20 Ward, R., *The postal history of Upper Wharfedale, Ilkley & Otley*. Publication No. 6, Yorkshire Postal History Society, Sheffield, 1972. p. 72.

21 *Ilkley Gazette*, 25 November 1977. p. 10.

22 Lukis, J.H., 1862. p. 209.

23 West View House was the home of Margaret Craig, the matron at Wells House Hotel. Dixon's Hall, later called Ilkley Hall, was built in 1825 for Joshua Dixon from Wakefield. The Dixon family then sold off the land around the edge of their estate for building plots. In 1859 the hall was used as a school by a Miss Adcock. In recent years it was the childhood home of the author, Gilly Cooper, and subsequently the offices of Spooner Engineering Ltd.

24 The name 'Crescent' is a puzzle. The building was in a straight terrace not a crescent, so perhaps the name was chosen for a sign or emblem. The crescent was a popular heraldic device and was, for example, part of the arms of the Percy family who had historic links with Ilkley. The name caused a great deal of confusion after the Crescent Hotel was opened in the town, and the owners of the West View property tried to distinguish it by changing the name to the Crescent House Hotel. This name was used until 1981 when it was sold and the new owner changed the name to 'Rombalds' – a return to its historic roots.

25 *Leeds Mercury*, 1 April 1843, p. 1.

26 *Leeds Mercury*, 26 August 1843, p. 4.

27 The vacant plot was not built on until 1879, thereby completing the row of three houses that now constitutes South View.

Chapter Five

Problems with Progress and Pallas

All the distractions of the Hydropathic Establishment could not keep Darwin from obsessing about Lyell's response to the *Origin*. 'From Lyell's letters he thinks favourably of it,' Darwin wrote to his younger botanist friend Hooker on 15 October:

> ...but seems staggered by the lengths to which I go. But if you go any considerable length in the admission of modification; I can see no possible means of drawing line, & saying here you must stop. Lyell is going to reread my Book, & yet I entertain hopes that he will be converted or *per*verted as he calls it.[1]

Such was Darwin's eagerness to win Lyell to the cause that, five days later, and without having yet received Lyell's reply to the long rebuttal letter of the 11th, Darwin wrote to him again. Darwin explained that he had been reading back over all of Lyell's letters on the *Origin*, and could now 'see in them evidence of fluctuation in the degree of credence you give to the theory; nor am I at all surprised at this, for many & many fluctuations I have undergone'.[2] The letter went on to offer supplementary thoughts on points raised in the letter of the 11th.

He returned to the question of why new species in the vicinity of America belong to the American type, even though their conditions of life are distinctly un-American (as in the Galapagos). Recall that he had rejected Lyell's suggestion that only thus could the creative power ensure that the new species would survive in the inevitable company of the old species. Darwin had pointed out that, since foreign species in America tend to have the competitive edge, the creative power's purposes would have been better served by casting the new species on other-than-American types. He now took their disagreement a step further, first by making a counter-argument on Lyell's behalf. Might not it be said in reply, Darwin ventured, that the creative power would nevertheless prefer the American type, since new species created to the other-than-American types would be too powerful – 'too well created so as to beat the aborigines', in Darwin's phrase – and so drive the old species to extinction instead of co-existing with them more or less stably? Darwin did not disguise his contempt for such impossible-to-refute theology. It seemed to him, he confessed, 'somehow a monstrous doctrine'.[3]

He also returned to the question of whether, to account for periodic advances in intelligence, one needs to suppose, as Lyell felt was necessary, the 'continued intervention of creative power'.

Darwin wrote that he had 'reflected a good deal' on Lyell's position, but could not persuade himself that Lyell was right. Once in motion, natural selection was sufficient to produce all the observed changes. Occasional meddling from a 'creative power' was a hypothesis of which Darwin had no need, he reckoned. Moreover, if the intervention hypothesis were needed, it would, Darwin emphasised again, 'make theory of nat. sel. valueless'. The whole point of the theory for Darwin – and what made it, in his eyes, such an impeccably Lyellian piece of science – was that it called upon only witnessable, regularly occurring natural causes in action around us now, as documented in the *Origin*. No creative interventions were needed, once the organismic basics (however they emerged) were in place. 'Grant a simple archetypal creature, like the Mud-fish or *Lepidosiren* [the scientific name for these air-breathing American fish], with the five senses & some vestige of mind,' Darwin explained to Lyell, '& I believe Natural Selection will account for production of every Vertebrate animal'.[4]

A letter from Hooker soon bore tantalisingly good news about Lyell, to judge from Darwin's reply (Hooker's letter does not survive). 'What you say about Lyell, pleases me exceedingly,' Darwin wrote back on 23 October:

I had not at all inferred from his letters that he had come so much round. I remember thinking above a year ago; that if I ever lived to see Lyell, yourself & [the anatomist Thomas Henry] Huxley come round, partly by my Book & partly by their own reflexions, I sh[oul]d feel that the subject was safe; & all the world might rail, but that ultimately the theory of Natural Selection (though no doubt imperfect in its present condition, & embracing many errors) would prevail. Nothing will ever convince me that three such men, with so much diversified knowledge, & so well accustomed to search for truth, could err greatly.[5]

Darwin had previously written to Huxley – like Hooker, a rising star in the younger generation, and already well-disposed toward Darwin – along similar lines the week before ('if on the whole, you & two or three others think that I am on the right road, I shall not care what the mob of naturalists think').[6] Before Darwin's time in Ilkley was through, he would receive testimonials from Hooker, Huxley and Lyell indicating their strong support for the theory, much to his relief and delight. But for now the greatest prize, Lyell, was playing hard to get – and on one topic, Man, would remain forever elusive.

No sooner had Darwin sent his deftly flattering letter to Hooker than a new letter from Lyell arrived, dated 22 October. Two topics especially were on Lyell's mind, one continuing an ongoing conversation, the other starting on something fresh. Lyell was still not convinced that natural selection on its own could accomplish all the extraordinary things that Darwin credited to it, most importantly the origin of Man. In Lyell's letter of the 4th, he had suggested that the 'same foreknowledge' that explained the creative power's preference for casting Galapagan species on the American type had to be generalised to 'the plans of Nature' overall. Suppose, wrote Lyell, that at the very beginning of life on Earth, the creative power had endowed 'a single primeval egg with the germs of all that was to be afterwards developed' – had programmed it, in other words, to unfold gradually the lineage of species that actually evolved. There would then be an explanation for the remarkable progression up the scale of life, culminating in Man, that Darwin and so many other naturalists believed they discerned in the fossil record. Lyell was famously dubious about the progressive pattern. But he nevertheless reckoned that

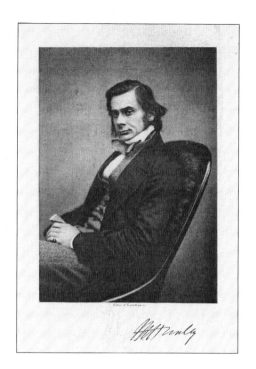

Thomas Henry Huxley (1825 – 95). 'His mind is as quick as a flash of lightning and as sharp as a razor,' Darwin later wrote of his anatomical ally, who by 1859 was already known for uncompromising – and hugely entertaining – scientific polemics.
(© National Portrait Gallery, London)

if, like Darwin, he believed in the pattern, and believed that natural selection had played a role in bringing it about, then he would need to suppose some kind of set-from-the-start, progressive, improving principle to have been working alongside natural selection, however high the intellectual cost of doing so – for, as Lyell made plain, such a principle would be, for the likes of Darwin and him, 'as mysterious & undefinable as "Creation"'.[7]

In the new letter, Lyell rehearsed these points, and then some. He argued that:

> ...unless there was an inherent 'tho for ages perhaps latent principle of improvement how evolve the Elephant & finally Man out of a Lepidosyren or even the much higher Ornithorhyncus [platypus]. Selection or breeding is merely giving the organism a free & fair chance of developing the inherent capacity. It is simply putting the acorn in the fittest soil... The appearance of Man viewed as progressive development views it, is in the organic world, I presume, the grandest & latest catastrophe... I care not for the term 'Creation' but I want something higher than 'selection', unless the latter divinity be supposed to have produced the primeval egg or seed or germ of the first great branches of the organic kingdom – in some ante-Cambrian epoch – To that power I must refer all the wonders of successive groups of species, more especially every step gained in organization & intelligence, generation [i.e. reproduction, including inheritance and variability – a core element of natural selection theory] being a very subordinate part of the machinery.[8]

In addition to affirming his views on the limits of natural selection theory when it came to evolutionary progress, Lyell in his letter of the 22nd opened up a new and quite different line of questioning. The subject was dogs, specifically whether the domesticated breeds of dog all trace back to one wild progenitor species or – as Darwin seems to suggest in the *Origin* – to more than one such species. For readers of the *Origin* today, the question does not stand out as among the more important ones addressed in the book. Darwin's main discussion appears in the difficult middle chapter on 'Hybridism', where he seeks to undermine the then-common notion that when organisms belonging to different species mate, the offspring are sterile so as, in Darwin's phrase, 'to prevent the confusion of all organic forms'. On this creationist view, the sterility of hybrids is yet another sign of the good design principles at work in the creation of species. Horses are kept horsey and donkeys donkeyish, for example, because the offspring of horse-donkey unions – mules – are kept sterile.[9]

In building up his argument against this view, Darwin at one point considers cases where hybrids *have* proved fertile. Among these cases are, he reckons, domesticated dogs. Darwin does not represent himself as going way out on a limb in supposing that dogs derive from more than one ancestral species. He credits the German naturalist Pyotr Simon Pallas (1741-1811) as author of the general 'doctrine… largely accepted by modern naturalists; namely, that most of our domestic animals have descended from two or more aboriginal species, since commingled by intercrossing'. On the Pallasian view favoured by Darwin, the fact that fertile offspring result no matter which dog breeds with which shows not that all dogs derive from a single common ancestral species, but rather that, as a result of domestication, several ancestral dog species independently lost their tendency to produce sterile offspring with each other.[10] (Domestication for Darwin was a process very disruptive of reproductive physiology; hence, in Darwin's view, the far greater variability found on farms than in nature. Modern science does not, in this matter as in many others, follow Darwin.)

In his letter, Lyell asked Darwin to expand on his few pages in the *Origin* on domesticated dogs. Thanks to new historical research, modern readers are in a much better position to understand quite why these pages disturbed Lyell so greatly. At stake was something far more consequential than getting the evolutionary origin of greyhounds and spaniels right. Throughout the 1840s and 1850s, debate about the origins of domesticated animals, and the bearing on this issue of their capacities for successful hybridization, had flourished as a major front – a kind of proxy theatre – for a politically explosive debate on the human races. Do all humans belong to one species, deriving from a common ancestral stock? Or does each race derive from its own ancestral species, independent of all the others? The answer had political moment because defenders of black slavery in the United States – the final holdout on slavery in the English-speaking world – were bent on portraying blacks as belonging to another, separate, sub-human species. That defence was almost traditional among the planters of the Southern states. But it had a new lease of scientific life with the rise in America of a new generation of sophisticated defenders. Where the anti-slavery, unity-of-man side of the debate was wont to argue, for example, that humans of every race can mate successfully with humans of every other race, thus demonstrating their common bond as members of a single species, the pro-slavery, 'pluralist' side responded with scepticism bolstered by statistics and experiments. Had anyone really looked to see, they asked, how successful were the results of mixed-race unions? Some of the pluralists' data suggested to them that mulattos – the offspring of white Europeans and blacks – were, true to their name (which derived from 'mule'), less fertile, and indeed that mulatto lineages soon became exhausted (again, modern science demurs). In a similar polemical vein, pluralists sought to throw doubt on the notion that only parents belonging to the same species could produce fertile offspring. Here, domesticated animals came to the fore, as subjects of experimental hybridization studies. They also featured as historical subjects, whose origins could be traced back to multiple, wild ancestors.[11]

Lyell and Darwin shared a commitment to a shared ancestry for the human races. Lyell had gone into print along such lines in his *Principles*.[12] As to Darwin's position, Lyell was in no doubt about it, since Darwin – whose extended family were unstinting supporters of the British anti-slavery campaign – had made plain his irritation with Lyell over the latter's kindly view toward the slavers he had met in America in the 1840s.[13] So Lyell fully expected that Darwin in the *Origin* would argue that all the domesticated varieties of a certain kind could be traced back to a single ancestral species. All the pigeons back to a single, ancestral pigeon species; all the dogs back to a single, ancestral dog species; and so on. And indeed, Darwin had made just that sort of unity case for pigeons, with an intellectual showstopper of an argument drawing on his own hybridization and related studies with domesticated pigeons in his garden at Down House in the late 1850s.[14] But with dogs he had gone for plurality, not unity – and Lyell did not know what to make of it, least of all when it came to Lyell and Darwin's common cause of giving the human races a common ancestry. Lyell wrote to Darwin:

> If I find myself perplexed with the distance between the European, Negro, Hottentot & Australian races & am told that they probably may have sprung from several indigenous stocks or species settled in remote & isolated regions which preceded all those now living & which by blending together gave origin to the diversity now observed. I feel instead of this being an explanation of my difficulty that it simply obscures all my ideas. Of course according to your system there was some common ancestor of all these races, as of the greyhound, pug, shepherd's dog &c. But how does Pallas' notion of several wild species being the ancestors in common of these races help us [?].... Whatever you yield in regard to the dog you will have to concede to every variable species of plant or animal (wild or cultivated) Man included.[15]

In Darwin's reply of 25 October, he dealt briefly with both the progress problem and the Pallas problem. On progress, Darwin drew Lyell's attention to an important distinction, between 'improvement' in the sense of species becoming better adapted to their respective conditions of life, and 'improvement' in the sense of species becoming more complexly organised and intelligent over the evolutionary long run. As Darwin explained, the theory of natural selection is in the first instance a theory of improvement in the former, adapting sense. Natural selection preserves and accumulates those inheritable variations which, chancing to arise, better fit species to their conditions. Sometimes it pays to stay simple, or even to get simpler – so there is no difficulty, on Darwin's theory, in explaining why some species are stubbornly primitive, and others derive from more complex ancestors. But sometimes it will pay to be more complex; and under these conditions, natural selection will preserve and accumulate variations tending toward greater complexity – 'and I can see no limit', Darwin added, 'to this process of improvement [,] without the intervention of any other & direct principle of improvement'. Some re-reading and reflection on the *Origin*'s first four chapters would, Darwin suggested, surely help ease Lyell's difficulties on this point.[16]

On the Pallas problem, Darwin admitted that the case for multiple ancestors for domesticated dogs was 'very hypothetical. Yet I certainly believe (but cannot here give reasons),' he went on, 'that the American domestic dogs have descended from at least 3 or 4 aboriginally distinct species, & that European dogs probably from several other species'. In Darwin's view, what kept this scenario from contradicting his general emphasis on common ancestry was that these several wild ancestors were themselves descended from a single ancestral stock. The big-picture story with dogs was thus one of divergence away from a common ancestor – exactly the story that the likes of Darwin and Lyell sought to tell about domesticated animal breeds generally, and about the human races as well. Yes, for the dogs, there was very probably this further, complicating, pluralist wrinkle to the story. But so what? 'It is', wrote Darwin, 'a curious, but not important subject for us: **we** believe that all canine species have descended from one parent; & the only question is whether the *whole* or only a part of the difference between our domestic breeds has arisen since man domesticated them'. He added, 'The Races of Man offer great difficulty: I do not think doctrine of Pallas, or that of Agassiz that there are several species of man, helps **us** in the least'.[17]

Mention of Agassiz underscored not just the human-racial resonances of this debate over dogs, but the human-political ones. Based at Harvard, the Swiss-born naturalist and geologist Louis Agassiz was the most powerful figure in the life sciences in the United States – and notorious, in Darwin's circles, for using that power to bolster the slave system there by backing a plural origin for the different human races. For Agassiz, these, in common with all plant and animal species, had been specially created in and for their own distinctive geographic zones of origination. The human races had come into being not as modified descendants of an ancestral stock but separately and exactly as we find them. In the past, Darwin had not hesitated to make plain the connection between this denial of genealogical connection and the maintenance of the American slave system. In 1850, in a letter remarking on 'Agassiz's Lectures in the U.S.', Darwin noted Agassiz's support there for 'the doctrine of several species, – much, I daresay, to the comfort of the slave-holding Southerns'.[18] But perhaps even Agassiz could be turned; he would be among the recipients of a presentation copy of the *Origin*, and also one of Darwin's Ilkley-composed letters of introduction.

Although Lyell let go (for the time being) on evolutionary progress, he remained concerned about the dogs. Hadn't Darwin needlessly given ammunition to the enemy in allowing for a plural origin for the dogs? 'I cannot help thinking', wrote Lyell in his reply to Darwin of 28 October, 'that by taking this concession, one which regards a variable species, about which we know most (little 'tho it be) an adversary may erect a battery against several of your principal rules, & in proportion as I am *per*verted I shall always feel inclined to withstand so serious a wavering'.[19] Darwin wrote back three days later, still unconcerned that the more complicated story one needed to tell for the origin of domesticated dogs made that story any less vindicating of his general theory than the less complicated story told for domesticated pigeons:

> Although the Hound – Greyhound & Bull-dog may possibly have descended from 3 distinct stocks, I am convinced that their present great amount of difference is mainly due to the same causes [i.e. selective breeding by humans], which have made the breeds of pigeons so different from each other, though these breeds of pigeons have all descended from **one** wild stock. So that the Pallasian doctrine, I look at, as of but quite secondary importance.[20]

We have no record of a reply from Lyell until weeks later, dated 21 November. Although short, it dealt entirely with the Pallas problem. 'The admission which I least like among your familiar illustrations,' he began, 'is that while the various pigeons have descended from one stock the dogs have come from two or more species'.[21] Darwin wrote back straight away. Undoubtedly, it would have been more convenient if the dog story had turned out to be as simple as the pigeon story. Alas, Nature had not been so obliging. 'I sh[oul]d infinitely prefer the theory of single origin in all cases', wrote Darwin, 'if facts would permit its reception'. But the facts in the dog case resisted that theory. Darwin explained that he found it very improbable, given the range of canine species available around the world for human domestication, and the resemblance between at least three domesticated breeds in America and some of the wild canines there, that just one species should have become the object of human efforts to domesticate dogs and breed new varieties, adapted to human needs and desires.[22]

Darwin wrote his reply on 23 November, the day before the official publication of the *Origin*. At the top of the letter he gave his address as 'Ilkley Wells' – the Wells House Hydro. But this was with a view to facilitating the arrival of Lyell's next letter. The 23rd was in fact Darwin's last day outside the hotel, in a house just down the road from it. Called North House, it had been the Darwin family's home since the middle of October. The whole of Darwin's side of the exchange with Lyell on domestication had been conducted from within North House, surrounded by many of the sights, sounds and – with the return of home cooking – smells and tastes of domestic life as usual.

Notes

1   C.D. to J.D. Hooker, 15 October [1859]; Correspondence, 7, p. 349, emphasis in original.

2   C.D. to Charles Lyell, 20 October [1859]; Correspondence, 7, p. 353.

3   C.D. to Charles Lyell, 20 October [1859]; Correspondence, 7, p. 353.

4   C.D. to Charles Lyell, 20 October [1859]; Correspondence, 7, p. 354. Darwin did not feel that he had to explain how basic organisms came into existence, any more than physicists had to explain how gravitation came into existence. As he put it in his letter to Lyell of the 11th: 'We must under present knowledge assume the creation of one or of a few forms, in same manner as [natural] philosophers assume the existence of a power of attraction, without any explanation'. C.D. to Charles Lyell, 11 October [1859]; Correspondence, 7, p. 345.

5   C.D. to J.D. Hooker, [23 October 1859], Correspondence, 7, p. 356.

6   C.D. to T.H. Huxley, 15 October [1859]; Correspondence, 7, p. 351.

7   Charles Lyell to C.D., 4 October 1859; Correspondence, 13, p. 411.

8   Charles Lyell to C.D., 22 October 1859; Correspondence, 13, p. 419.

9   Darwin, C., *On the Origin of Species* (John Murray, London 1859), p. 245. Darwin also remarked briefly on the multiple origins of domesticated dogs in the first chapter. (pp. 18-20)

10   Darwin, C., *On the Origin of Species* (John Murray, London 1859), pp. 253–254.

11   Desmond, A., and Moore, J., *Darwin's Sacred Cause: Race, Slavery and the Quest for Human Origins* (Allen Lane, London 2009), esp. chs 6–8.

12   Lyell directed readers to other writers who had furnished 'convincing proofs that the varieties of form, colour, and organization of different races of men, are perfectly consistent with the generally received opinion, that all the individuals of the species have originated from a single pair; and while

they exhibit in man as many diversities of a physiological nature, as appear in any other species, they confirm also the opinion of the slight deviation from a common standard of which a species is capable'. Lyell, C., *Principles of Geology* (Penguin, London 1997), p. 230.

13 Desmond, A., and Moore, J., *Darwin's Sacred Cause: Race, Slavery and the Quest for Human Origins* (Allen Lane, London 2009), ch. 7, esp. pp. 180–181.

14 Darwin, C., *On the Origin of Species* (John Murray, London 1859), pp. 20–29. Our interpretation of the Ilkley correspondence over domesticated dogs is indebted to Desmond and Moore's pioneering discussion. Desmond, A., and Moore, J., *Darwin's Sacred Cause: Race, Slavery and the Quest for Human Origins* (Allen Lane, London 2009), pp. 311–313.

15 Charles Lyell to C.D., 22 October 1859; Correspondence, 13, pp. 418–419.

16 C.D. to Charles Lyell, 25 October [1859]; Correspondence, 7, p. 358. On Darwin on evolutionary progress, see Radick, G., 'Two explanations of evolutionary progress', *Biology and Philosophy*, 2000; 15: 475–491.

17 C.D. to Charles Lyell, 25 October [1859]; Correspondence, 7, pp. 357–358, emphases in original.

18 Desmond, A., and Moore, J., *Darwin's Sacred Cause: Race, Slavery and the Quest for Human Origins* (Allen Lane, London 2009), ch. 9, quotation from letter on p. 242.

19 Charles Lyell to C.D., 28 October 1859; Correspondence, 7, p. 363, emphasis in original.

20 C.D. to Charles Lyell, 31 [October 1859]; Correspondence, 7, p. 364, emphasis in original.

21 Charles Lyell to C.D., 21 November 1859; Correspondence, 7, p. 384.

22 C.D. to Charles Lyell, 23 November [1859]; Correspondence, 7, p. 392. A reviewer of Desmond and Moore's book, John Carey, picked out the quoted phrase from Darwin's letter as an important sign that, in Darwin's case, the influence of politics over science had a limit (*Sunday Times*, 25 January 2009).

Chapter Six

North House

Once Emma had decided to join Charles in Ilkley, he set about finding a house to let near to Wells House. The search did not take long. The hotel manager, Mr Strachan, was well aware that Mr Marshall Hainsworth had houses to let in Wells Terrace. One of his houses had been occupied by Dr Rischanek after his dismissal from Wells House and, much to the annoyance of Dr Smith, Rischanek resumed independent hydropathic practice, using the baths at White Wells.[1] As it turned out, he had little personal following and after a short time he abandoned his practice and withdrew from the Ilkley hydropathic scene.

Marshall Hainsworth and his brothers, Jonathan and Timothy, were stonemasons and all had worked on the building of Wells House.[2] In 1857, they turned their attention to the erection of a block of three houses, to be called Wells Terrace, for their father – Timothy Hainsworth Snr, a farmer at Burley Woodhead near Ilkley.[3] On completion, one of the houses was occupied by Marshall, with his wife Elizabeth, young daughter Ann, and a couple of servants, along with Marshall's brother Jonathan and occasional lodgers. The other houses were let on a short-term basis. Darwin learnt that one of these houses, North House, was vacant, so he approached Dr Smith about living 'out of establishment'. This proved to be a less straightforward matter.

Dr Smith had strong feelings about his patients being 'in the establishment' and no doubt produced a well-rehearsed homily against residence in lodgings when approached by Darwin. Smith held the view that hydropathic patients should be under the immediate and constant supervision of a doctor:

> This is an advantage they cannot enjoy if he [the patient] resides at a distance, and only makes a daily visit at the stated time. Precious minutes which may make the difference of life and death are not wasted in sending for him. He is on the spot, and ever ready with the resources of his art, at all hours of the day or night. Urgent symptoms can be met as they arise, and pressing danger be averted without delay. Every stage of disease can be minutely watched and promptly treated with appropriate remedies; and the effect of treatment, immediate or subsequent, can be accurately determined.[4]

In spite of Dr Smith's alarmist arguments against 'out-patient' treatment, Darwin's request to move off-site must have met with at least grudging approval, and he made immediate

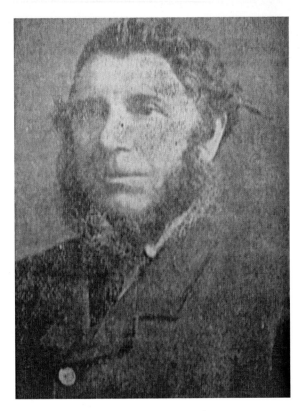

Marshall Hainsworth, owner of Wells Terrace. A mason by trade, Hainsworth helped to build Wells House Hotel before turning his attention to the three houses that formed Wells Terrace. A quiet, thrifty man, he acquired a good deal of other properties in Ilkley and amassed a considerable fortune before his death in 1897. (*Ilkley Gazette*/Alex Cockshott)

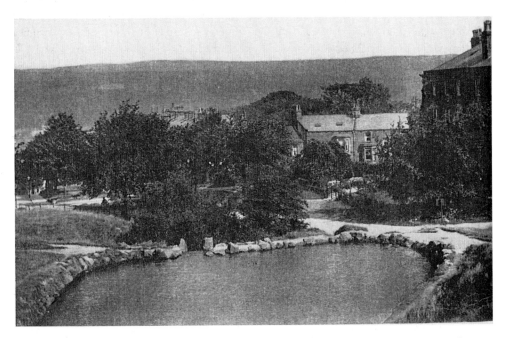

Hainsworth's Pond with Wells Terrace on the right. The houses ahead are those of South View and were across Cross Beck Bridge Road (now Crossbeck Road).

arrangements to rent the house from Mr Hainsworth. Thus, on Friday 14 October, Darwin, though still at Wells House, wrote a letter to his son William bearing the address 'North House, Wells Terrace, Ilkley, Otley, Yorkshire':

My dear William

On Monday they all come from Barlaston to the above address & I leave the Establishment.[5] The House is at the foot of a rocky, turfy rather steep half-mountain. It would be nice with fine weather; but now looks dismal. There are nice excursions & fine walks for those that can walk. The Water Cure has done me much good; but I fell down on Sunday morning & sprained my ancle (sic), & have not been able to walk since & this has greatly interfered with the treatment.

It is a curious life here: we sit down 60 or 70 to our meals, & in the evening, there is either singing, or acting (which they do capitally) or proverbs &c.- I have got amongst a nice set, & get on very comfortably & idly. The newspaper, a little novel reading, the Baths & loitering kills the day in a very wholesome manner. Did you ever hear of the American game of Billiards: <five lines excised> There are some splendid players here who often make breaks of 20, 30, & 40. These good players never play anything but the American game.- I shall miss the Billiard Table when I leave here & go into our House which is <incomplete>

Who were these sixty or seventy fellow diners? Darwin discloses the identity of only a few. Apart from his lady friend, Mary Butler, he only mentions one other party – the Cromptons. 'Poor Mr. Crompton who has just lost his wife, is here, & the old Lady who seems very nice: I have not seen the invalid daughter'.[6] John Gilbert Crompton, Lord of the Manor of Bonsall in Derbyshire and a former Mayor of Chesterfield, was acquainted with Darwin's cousin William Fox. Crompton's wife, Millicent, had died very recently – on 4 October 1859, hence Darwin's sympathetic tone. The remaining guests are anonymous, but we can make some attempt at describing the clientele.

The national census of 1861 gives a list of people staying at Wells House in April of that year, and assuming it to be representative, we can create a picture of the guests likely to have been present with Darwin. While the census return gives the visitors' ages and occupations, we can only surmise as to why they were there. Using this approach, his fellow guests probably included several over-wrought businessmen needing time to unwind, bored men and women 'of property' with too much time on their hands; one or two senior civil servants on furlough from India; churchmen seeking rest (and re-creation?); a few single 'gentlewomen' whose only illness was a want of love; war-weary Army officers trying to forget and confused old gentlemen trying to remember; and a disillusioned medical practitioner or two seeking help from the unorthodox.[7] The age profile of the guests is interesting. Although they range from eight to sixty-seven years, the distribution was skewed towards younger adults such that the median age was thirty-four and a half years. To the modern reader this seems surprisingly young, but it should be borne in mind that visitors to a Hydro had 'complaints' and not necessarily diseases.

Whether it was entirely chance, or Darwin's choice, he ended up in 'a nice set'. Surprisingly, given his anti-social reputation, he enjoyed the home-spun entertainments on offer in the evenings: the singing, acting and the recitations. As with Moor Park, it appears that Wells House brought out a different Darwin – an extrovert Darwin who responded to the company of young women and felt comfortable with convivial men; a version of the man largely unknown to his scientific associates and his correspondents. He did, however, greatly miss the company of his family and he was eager to be reunited with them at North House. His only slight regret seems to be that he would miss the billiard table.

Billiards was very much part of Darwin's 'wholesome' days at the Hydro. He was introduced to the game as a young man and played when he visited Woodhouse, the home of family friends, the convivial William Mostyn Owen and his two pretty daughters. At one time Darwin was infatuated with the flirtatious Fanny Owen, and she teased him over many things, including billiards. In a letter written to him when he was a student at Cambridge, she declared, 'I am shocked to inform you that I have not yet learn't to play at Billiards… but it is not my fault I assure you, for I can get nobody to give me some lesson's… so I suppose I must trust to fate for a master or wait till you come'.[8] Apparently, Darwin remedied the situation on his next visit to Woodhouse and gave Fanny the billiards lessons she sought. Eight months later, she wrote, 'Not one game of Billiards have I had since I play'd with you. I can get nobody to play with & am afraid for want of practice shall forget all my fine strokes'.[9]

Certainly, Darwin must have forgotten all his fine strokes by the time he resumed the game. It is likely that his next chance to play billiards in any sustained fashion was while undergoing water cure treatment at Moor Park. In May 1858, he wrote to his son William, 'I have been playing a good deal at Billiards, & have lately got up to my play & made some splendid strokes!'[10] Darwin's letters to William around this time are full of anecdotes and good humour. We can now see that it was natural for him to reveal the relaxed, non-academic side of his character by reference to billiards. On another visit to Moor Park, in February 1859, he tells William of his progress, or lack of it, and it is apparent that they are on the look-out for a billiard table for Down House:

Nor can I get up to my old standard in Billiards. There is a young Irishman here, who plays capitally and gives me lessons: he always is hitting his own ball on one side, but Dr Lane says that if I take to that I shall never learn, so that it is hard work to settle between my masters. It is horrid that one cannot play on Sundays & makes the day very long for I like watching the others. The other day there was an advertisement of 11 ft Thurston table at Dickensons for 17 guineas; I wonder whether that was the one you saw: if not it is disgusting that I did not advertise.[11]

Less than two weeks later, a brand new billiard table was installed at Down House. It cost the princely sum of £53 18s, and Darwin must have felt some pangs of conscience over spending such a large amount on a mere frivolity, because he used some of the proceeds of the sale of the Wedgwood family's slate reliefs that they had inherited, and his father's gold watch, to pay for the table.[12] Shortly afterwards, the Darwins were visited by Henry Wedgwood ('Uncle Harry') and his children Louisa and John. Following their visit, Darwin again writes to William about the billiards:

I have thought that you would like to hear about Table. John thinks it a very good one. He is a goodish player, & one day made 33 points without a break or a fluke. – He is a much better player than I, yet I somehow generally beat him; I beat him two games running of 30. – You never saw anything like Georgy & the billiards; I think on Saturday he played for 10 hours; one game of a 100 with Parslow took them, I think, two hours. We have bought a stunning Book on Billiards, costing 21s., & it has nearly 200 diagrams of various strokes & accounts of famous games. Altogether the Table has been a splendid purchase.[13]

The billiard table at Wells House was, therefore, a big attraction for Darwin. He would have played some of the time, but also sat around watching others play American Billiards. The American game was played with four balls, two white and two red, and used only four pockets, but otherwise was like the English game where players earned points by pocketing balls, going in-off, or by making canons which were called 'caroms'.[14] After 17 October, Darwin's visits to the billiard room would be strictly curtailed.

Darwin and the family moved into North House. Who exactly constituted 'the family' in Ilkley is a matter of some conjecture. Darwin wrote to Lady Drysdale (of Moor Park), 'I staid in the establishment for a fortnight and then took a House and all my family are here'.[15] William (aged twenty), however, was up at Christ's College, Cambridge, and George (aged fourteen) was a boarder at Clapham Grammar School. The 'family', therefore, comprised his wife and Henrietta (aged sixteen), Elizabeth (aged twelve), and probably Francis (aged eleven), Leonard (aged nine) and Horace (aged eight). Certainly, Etty and Lizzy were in Ilkley – Emma records their body weights (7st 9lb and 6st 5lb respectively) in her journal on 19 October, and mentions them (but no one else) when they depart.[16] If all the children apart from William and George visited Ilkley, they are unlikely to have travelled without the children's governess and Parslow, the butler, might have accompanied them. No reference to their presence in Ilkley has come to light.

Just as the make-up of the family group is sketchy, so the domestic arrangements are unrecorded. Who did the cooking? Surely, it was not all done by Emma. Mrs Hainsworth might have provided some cooking, she was noted for her 'kindly consideration and attention to the comforts of her guests', or she might have provided a servant as part of the rental arrangements.[17] It is possible that some meals were taken in Wells House. Joining Charles and his 'set' around the dining table would have given Emma the opportunity to make the acquaintance of Mary Butler. At the end of October, Emma wrote to William, 'Miss Butler your father's friend of Moor Park is gone which is a great loss to us as she is very pleasant & lively & kind'.[18] Emma's sentiments regarding the younger woman speak volumes for the confidence she had in her relationship with Charles.

As to how the family occupied their time in Ilkley, we know that they went on an excursion to Bolton Abbey, and there may have been other 'drives' organised from Wells House stables.[19] Popular destinations included Barden Tower, the Strid Woods and Burnsall higher up Wharfedale, and Denton, Farnley and Almscliff Crags down the valley, while longer excursions to Haworth, Fountains Abbey or Harrogate were also on offer. One excursion that Darwin might have been expected to take was a visit to a relative, Francis Rhodes Darwin, who lived at Kirkskill Hall, Arthington. Although a 'Darwin' in name, his kinship was a distant one. Born Francis Rhodes, he married Charlotte Maria Darwin Cooper, a remote cousin of Charles Darwin, in 1849. Rhodes took the name 'Darwin' in 1850 under the terms of the will of his brother-in-law, Robert Alvey Darwin, who died young (aged twenty) in Madeira, and whose estate Rhodes inherited. Despite acquiring the splendid Elston Hall in Nottingham through this inheritance, Francis continued to occupy the Rhodes family home, Kirkskill Hall (later called Creskeld Hall), a largely nineteenth-century house constructed around remnants of its medieval origins. Charles Darwin, however, chose not to visit. He wrote, 'I find that Mr. Rhoades (sic) Darwin lives about 10 miles off, near Arthington Stn. at a very nice place – I shd. like to call there, but shall not have strength or spirits'.[20]

A similar excursion that Darwin could have taken, but chose to decline, was a visit to Burley-in-Wharfedale suggested by Reverend Charles Kingsley, the academic and author. Although best known as the writer of the *Water Babies*, Kingsley was an enthusiastic natural historian. In 1854, Kingsley met Darwin on one of his occasional visits to a meeting of the Linnaean Society in London.[21] Knowing that Darwin was staying in Ilkley, Kingsley wrote to him suggesting that he might like to meet Mr W. E. Forster who lived at 'Wharfeside' in Burley, but Darwin politely rejected the notion.[22] Forster was a wealthy mill-owner, Member of Parliament and educational reformer, and a long-standing friend of Charles Kingsley. Kingsley visited the Forsters in 1858, and the contrast between his rural parish in Hampshire and the Northern industrial village of Burley struck him forcibly. 'I am in a state of bewilderment,' he wrote home, 'such machinery as no tongue can describe, about three acres of mills, and a whole village of people, looking healthy, rosy and happy'.[23] Over 60 per cent of households in Burley had at least one member working in Forster's Greenholme Mills, so Kingsley's observations spoke well of the working conditions in these particular mills.[24]

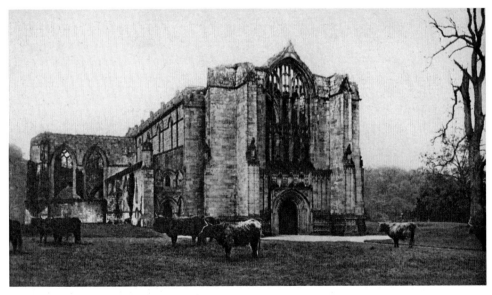

Bolton Priory (more commonly, but incorrectly, called 'Bolton Abbey'). In her journal, Emma Darwin records a visit to Bolton Abbey on 31 October 1859. Although much of it is in ruin, there has been a church in the nave of the Priory since the Dissolution, the Church of St Mary and St Cuthbert. The incumbent in 1859 was the Reverend John Umpleby although he no doubt left the job of guiding the Darwin party around the building to the verger.

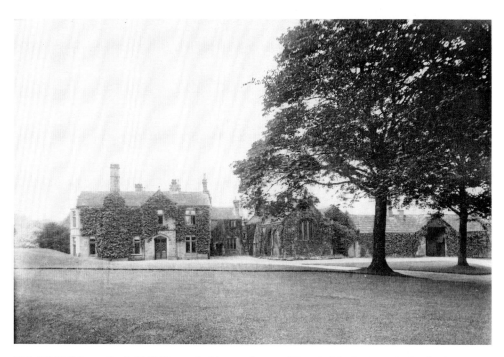

Kirkskill Hall (later Creskeld Hall) near Arthington, home of Francis Rhodes Darwin. (By kind permission of Leeds Civic Trust and Leeds Library and Information Services, www.leodis.net)

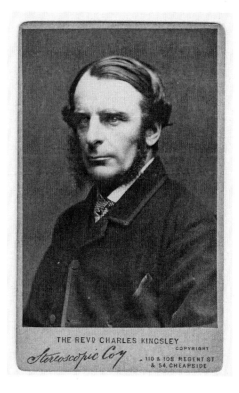

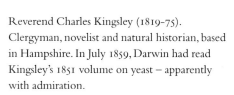

Reverend Charles Kingsley (1819-75). Clergyman, novelist and natural historian, based in Hampshire. In July 1859, Darwin had read Kingsley's 1851 volume on yeast – apparently with admiration.
(© National Portrait Gallery, London)

If a carriage excursion did not appeal, the moor was on the doorstep and, when weather permitted, there could have been family walks up to White Wells or up the Keighley Road with its splendid views over the valley. The weather, however, was not kind to the visitors. Darwin was quite right about Wells Terrace being 'dismal' in the grey days of autumn. North House had a spectacular view from its upper windows, but in the steady drizzle that often prevails in October in the Wharfe Valley, the prospect would be dank and dull. Being north-facing, the rooms too were gloomy and prone to coldness. In later years, Etty recalled her time in Ilkley, 'It was bitterly cold, he [her father] was extremely ill and suffering, the lodgings were uncomfortable, and I look back on it as a time of frozen misery'.[25]

Misery was the tone of a letter Darwin wrote to William just six days after taking up residence at North House, 'Here is a dreadful wet day – no baths, no nothing, & all the patients half dead with ennui'.[26] On the same day (23 October), he wrote to Hooker, 'The Doctor has brought out by wet bandages such an eruption & inflammation on my legs, that I cannot move; but it has done my stomach truly wonderful good'.[27] Two days later Darwin comments again on his legs, 'I am terribly lame with inflamed leg (what the Water-cure Doctors call a severe crisis) & this makes my hand-writing rather worse even than usual'.[28] He tells Hooker, 'I have been very bad lately; having had an awful "crisis" one leg swelled like elephantiasis – eyes almost closed up – covered with rash and fiery boils; but they tell me it will surely do me much good. – it was like living in Hell'.[29]

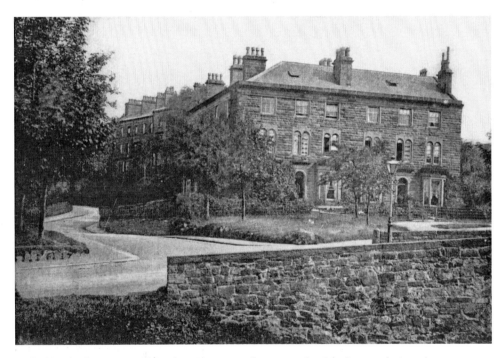

Wells Terrace. The two west-facing houses are seen, the one on the right (nearest the moor) was occupied by Marshall Hainsworth and his family. In 1859, and subsequently for many years thereafter, the house on the left and a third, north-facing house entered from Cross Beck Bridge Road, were let to visitors.

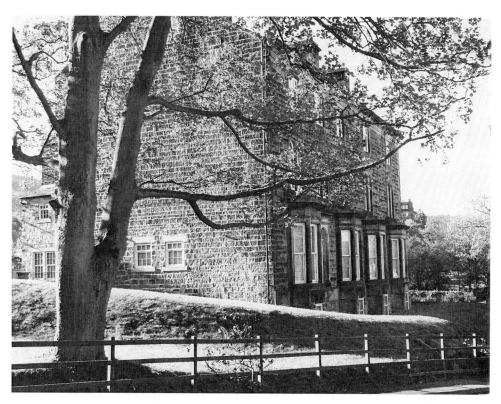

North and east-facing aspects of Wells Terrace, 2006. The apartments are now known as Hillside Court. A corner of Wells House can be seen over the trees behind.

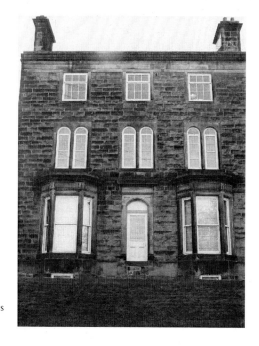

The former North House, Wells Terrace, 2006. The entrance door has been sealed and the steps leading up to it removed.

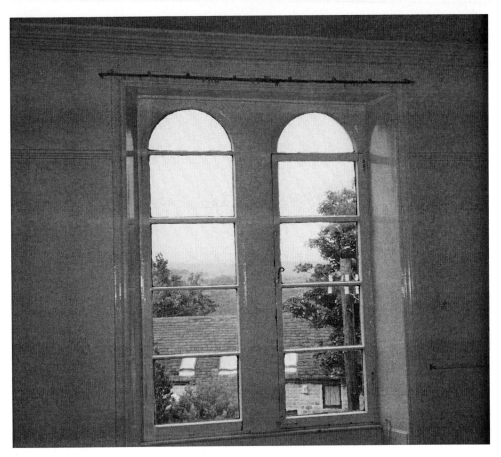

View from a first floor bedroom in the former North House, taken shortly before refurbishment in 1999. The upper part of a new house across Crossbeck Road is seen. In Darwin's time, this room would have had an uninterrupted view over the Wharfe Valley. (Kathryn Emmott)

One of the chief aims of hydropathy was to induce a 'crisis', and Darwin had heard much about it from Dr Gully:

> Whenever an organ or series of organs, in the state of morbid excitement which is present in acute and chronic disease, is placed, by art, in a condition to cast off that excitement, the act is announced by a change in some other organ, or organs. This change is a crisis… But as this change never takes place until the organ first diseased has cast off its morbid excitement, the change alluded to, i.e. the crisis, does not itself relieve the former but is a signal that it has relieved itself. It is for this reason that a crisis of some sort is desirable; it is an evidence of good having been affected.[30]

Gully described various forms of crisis. The most common was an eruption of the skin, but it could also be expressed by a fever, or through the lower bowel or kidneys – the usual routes for 'purgation'. The changes in the skin were usually mild; Gully described an efflorescence, a simple redness, or a rash of small pimples.

Occasionally, however, the patient had 'a crisis of boils'. To the orthodox medical practitioner such a term raised an alarming prospect. After the first edition of Gully's book, a number of eminent practitioners took up their pens to abuse Gully and his methods. One anonymous doctor wrote, 'the water cure will flourish until some person of note is crippled by a rheumatic fever or dead from a carbuncle'. In later editions of his book, Gully rose to counter such misguided claims. He pointed out that the 'water-boil' was quite different from the boils and carbuncles known to orthodox practitioners. The former were simple transudations of fluid into the skin causing localised swellings, whereas the latter were collections of pus which could spread and give rise to potentially fatal complications. These purulent boils and carbuncles were not a consequence of hydropathy. Gully also emphasised that the 'crisis of boils' was uncommon, 'Of upwards of 500 patients who have been under treatment at Malvern, not more than 22 have had an eruption of boils… But we can truthfully aver, that not one of these was deprived of an hour's sleep, nor debarred the usual exercise and diet for a single day'.[31] This was patently not Darwin's experience under the care of Dr Smith.

On the 16 November, Darwin gave a detailed summary of the course of his illness while in Ilkley to his cousin:

> I doubt whether Dr Smith would have suited you: they all say he is very careful in bad illness; but he constantly gives me impression, as if he cared very much for the Fee & very little for the patient. – I like the place very much, & the children have enjoyed it much & it has done my wife good; it did Etty good at first, but she has gone back again. – I have had a series of calamities; first a sprained ancle, & then badly swollen whole leg and face; much rash & a frightful succession of Boils – 4 or 5 at once, I have felt quite ill - & have little faith in this "unique crisis" as the Doctor calls it, doing me much good. I cannot now walk a step from bad boil on knee. We have been here above 6 week, & I feel worse than when I came; so that I am not in cheerful frame of mind… We shall stay about a fortnight longer here; & possibly though not probably I may stay a week or so still longer in Establishment; but it will depend on how I feel.[32]

Two days after this litany of medical disasters, Darwin continued in despondent mood, 'I am feeling very unwell today & this note is badly, perhaps hardly intelligibly expressed'.[33] His mood would not be improved by the departure of his family.[34] They chose a remarkably auspicious day on which to move, quitting North House on Thursday 24 November, and leaving Darwin, now returned to Wells House, to wrestle alone with his own particular 'crisis' – the crisis of publication.

Notes

1   *Leeds Mercury*, 1 May 1858. p. 1.

2   'Death of Marshall Hainsworth', *Ilkley Gazette*, 10 April 1897.

3   Timothy Hainsworth of Wood Cottage, Burley, purchased the land, originally forming part of the Cow Pastures, from the Inclosure Commissioners for England and Wales on 1 January 1857, Memorial TS/68/94, West Riding Registry of Deeds, Wakefield. Building of the block of three houses to be called Wells Terrace commenced shortly afterwards and was completed by early 1858.

Timothy Hainsworth remained the owner, but the property was occupied by Marshall Hainsworth and his tenants.

4   Lukis, J.H., 1862. p. 217.

5   Emma Darwin went to visit her brother, Francis (Frank) Wedgwood, who lived at Barlaston in Staffordshire on 7 October before journeying on to Ilkley on 17 October. Emma Darwin's diary 1859 (see http://darwin-online.org.uk/EmmaDiaries.html)

6   C.D. to W.D. Fox, 16 November 1859, Correspondence; 7, p. 377.

7   In the 1861 return for Wells House, a Dr James Wilson is listed among the twenty-two visitors. This was the same James Wilson who introduced the water cure to Malvern. Wilson also paid occasional visits to Ben Rhydding, and it was on one such visit (on the 8 January 1867) that he was found dead in his chair close to a tepid bath. (Grierson, J., *Dr Wilson and his Malvern Hydro*, Cora Weaver, Malvern: 1998, p. 97).

8   F.M. Owen, to C.D., 9 March 1828; Correspondence, 1, p. 53.

9   F.M. Owen to C.D. 26 October 1828; Correspondence, 1, p. 69.

10 C.D. to W.E. Darwin, 3 May 1858; Correspondence, 7, p. 87.

11 C.D. to W.E. Darwin, 13 February 1859; Correspondence, 7, p. 248.

12 C.D. to G. H. Darwin, 24 February 1859; Correspondence, 7, p. 251.

13 C.D. to W.E. Darwin 14 March 1859; Correspondence, 7, p. 263.

14 'Carom' was an abbreviation of '*carambole*' – the French term for this stroke at billiards.

15 C.D. to Lady Drysdale, 22 or 29 October 1859; Correspondence, 13, Supplement p. 416 and footnote 4, p. 417.

16 Emma Darwin's Diary 19 October 1859; http://darwin-online.org.uk/EmmaDiaries.html

17 'Death of Mrs Hainsworth', *Ilkley Gazette*. 30 April 1904.

18 Emma Darwin to W.E. Darwin, October 1959 (Cambridge University Library, DAR 210.6) See footnote 3, Correspondence, 7, p. 332.

19 The visit to Bolton Abbey took place on Monday 31 October. Emma Darwin's Diary, http://darwin-online.org.uk/EmmaDiaries.html.

20 C.D. to W.D. Fox, 16 November 1859; Correspondence, 7, p. 377, and www.leodis.net (Leeds photographic archive – Creskeld Hall). With the death of Robert Alvey Darwin, Francis Rhodes became head of the Elston Hall branch – the senior line, of the Darwin family. See C.D. to W.D. Fox, 8 July 1861; Correspondence, 9, p. 204, footnote 8.

21 Colloms, B., *Charles Kingsley: The Lion of Eversley* (Constable, London: 1975) p. 185.

22 The letter first suggesting the meeting with Forster is missing but can be implied from C.D.'s reply on 30 November 1859; Correspondence, 7, p. 407.

23 Colloms, B., 1975. p. 231.

24 Warwick, Margaret and D., *Eminent Victorians: The Forsters of Burley-in-Wharfedale*. (Burley-in-Wharfedale Local History Group Publications, 1994) p.20.

25 Litchfield, H., *Emma Darwin: A Century of Family Letters* (John Murray, London: 1915) vol. 2, p. 172.

26 C.D. to W.E. Darwin, 23 October – 20 November 1859; Correspondence, 7, p. 355.

27 C.D. to J.D. Hooker, 23 October 1859; Correspondence, 7, p. 336.

28 C.D. to Charles Lyell, 25 October 1859; Correspondence, 7, p. 358.

29 C.D. to J.D. Hooker, 27 October or 3 November 1859; Correspondence, 7, p. 362.

30 Gully, J.B., *The Water Cure in Chronic Disease*. Ninth edition. (Simpkin, Marshall, & Co., London: 1863) p. 448.

31 J.B. Gully 1863, pp. 444-447.

32 C.D. to W.D. Fox, 16 November 1859; Correspondence, 7, p. 377.

33 C.D. to W.B. Carpenter 18 November 1859; Correspondence, 7, p. 379.

34 Leaving Ilkley on 24 November, according to her diary, Emma 'with Etty and Lizzy' stayed that night in Manchester. On the 25th they travelled to Shrewsbury where they stayed until 6 December, travelling back to Down via London. (Emma Darwin's Diary, http://darwin-online.org.uk/EmmaDiaries.html).

Chapter Seven

Smoothing the Way

Well before publication day, Darwin had used the power of the pen – and the Ilkley Post Office – to help the *Origin* on its journey among the scientific elite. His correspondence with Hooker and Huxley, already discussed, shows signs of the wider campaign being waged. Writing to them from the Wells House Hydro on 15 October, Darwin had pumped them for names and addresses of foreign naturalists whose cast of mind was sufficiently theoretical – 'philosophical', in the terminology of the day – to be worth cultivating. Would it, Darwin asked Hooker, 'be any good to send copy of my Book to [the French botanist Joseph] Decaisne? And do you know any philosophical Botanist on Continent, who reads English & cares for such subjects? … How about [the botanist Nils Johan] Anders**s**?on in Sweden?'[1] From Huxley, Darwin requested the addresses of Joachim Barrande, a French-born, Prague-based palaeontological writer; Karl Theodor Ernst von Siebold, a German zoologist and comparative anatomist; and Alexandr Andreevich Keyserling, a Russian all-rounder in geology and natural history. 'Can you tell me,' Darwin added, 'of any good and *speculative* foreigners to whom it would be worth while to send copies of my Book 'on origin of species'… I sh[oul]d like to send a few about; but how many I can afford I know not yet till I hear what price Murray affixes'.[2]

Rather than wait for Murray, Darwin wrote to him that same day, explaining that in order to 'regulate' the number of presentation copies of the *Origin*, he needed to know the book's trade price as well as the charge Murray would rightly levy for the beyond-the-norm corrections requested on the proofs. At present, Darwin went on, he was reckoning on purchasing seventy copies (above the twelve that Murray was providing free-of-charge), with twenty-nine to be sent 'to almost every part of world to those who have assisted me, viz. Europe, N. America, India, Australia &c. &c.'[3] Murray's reply did not arrive until 3 November, but proved worth the wait. It carried not only the information on price that Darwin sought, and the good news that Murray would not charge extra for the proof changes, but the even better news that a specimen copy of the *Origin* was en route that same day. 'I have received your kind note & the copy,' Darwin immediately wrote back. 'I am *infinitely* pleased & proud at the appearance of my child'.[4] Now it was time to prepare the other recipients.

We do not have all the letters that Darwin wrote from Ilkley in advance of the arrival of his 'child' in its new homes; in the end over eighty presentation copies were sent.[5] The letters that survive – together with the ones we can infer from surviving responses – fall into roughly four

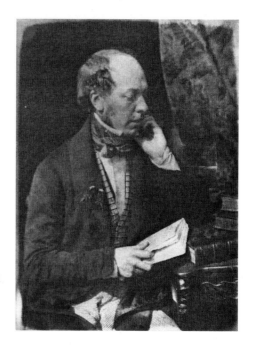

John Murray (1808-92). Darwin's publisher, who became head of the family firm in 1843, achieved considerable success in the firm's chosen niches of travel, history, biography and memoirs. (© National Portrait Gallery, London)

groups. First, there were the ones to his family. In his 16 November letter to his Cheshire cousin Fox, detailing Darwin's Ilkley health 'calamities' – the sprained ankle and so on – Darwin warned Fox that, if he hadn't already received it, he would:

> ...very soon receive my weariful book on Species. I naturally believe it mainly includes the truth, but you will not at all agree with me. – Dr. Hooker, whom I consider one of best judges in Europe, is complete convert, & he thinks Lyell is likewise. Certainly, judging from Lyell's letters to me on subject, he is deeply staggered.—'[6]

Health calamities notwithstanding, Darwin was at that moment deep in debate with Lyell on the origin of domesticated dogs and whether Darwin's advocacy of multiple wild ancestors contradicted his general theory, and the anti-slavery politics that went with it. It turned out that Lyell wasn't the only one to feel concerned. Another was Darwin's older sister, the passionately anti-slavery Caroline. In his reply to her, around 21 November, Darwin wrote both of his astonishment – and, obviously, delight – 'that you care as much for my Book as you seem to do', and of his concern that, given the difficulties she and Lyell had reported with the discussion on dogs, he really ought to have expressed himself more clearly. Darwin made plain to Caroline what he had written to Lyell; all the domesticated dogs trace back to a single ancient species, albeit – and here dog breeds were different from human races – via a number of distinct wild species. There was no contradiction, only complication.[7]

Yet another older sibling, his brother Erasmus, wrote a couple of days later to say how much he too had liked the book. Long-ago letters home from Erasmus had fired Charles' youthful enthusiasm for science by describing the chemical lectures the older boy had attended as a medical student at Cambridge University.[8] Now, Erasmus indicated, Charles had returned the favour. 'For myself I really think it is the most interesting book I ever read', wrote Erasmus, '& can only compare it to the first knowledge of chemistry, getting into a new world or rather behind the scenes'. What impressed Erasmus especially, he went on, were the geographical proofs, such as the commonalities Darwin brought out between island and mainland fauna. Where Lyell had cast doubt on those proofs, querying the neglected role of divine foreknowledge in stamping the two fauna with a single type, Erasmus regarded the proofs as surplus to need. 'In fact the a priori reasoning is so entirely satisfactory to me,' he wrote, 'that if the facts won't fit in, why so much the worse for the facts is my feeling'. Erasmus was not in fact feeling very fit himself at the moment – something he made light of in closing: 'My ague has left me in such a state of torpidity that I wish I had gone thro' the process of natural selection'.[9]

A second group of *Origin* recipients corresponded with from Ilkley were the English naturalists in his immediate circle – the ones close enough to Darwin to have known beforehand what kind of theory the book would promote. Hooker, Huxley and Lyell were the main figures here, of course. But there was also someone much less well known to Darwin personally. Famous today as the 'co-discoverer' of natural selection, Alfred Russel Wallace was then an uncelebrated specimen collector and occasional writer on philosophical natural history, eking out a living in the Malay Archipelago. Yet more than anyone else, it was Wallace who pushed Darwin into writing the *Origin*. For it was Darwin's alarmed discovery in June 1858 that Wallace had independently developed a similar theory of evolution that prompted Darwin to abandon a voluminous, for-experts-only, evolutionary treatise in favour of a popular 'abstract' for rapid publication. Long and demanding though it was, the *Origin* was that abstract. 'If you are so inclined,' Darwin wrote to Wallace on 13 November, 'I sh[oul]d very much like to hear your general impression of the Book as you have thought so profoundly on subject & and in so nearly same channel with myself… Remember it is only an abstract & very much condensed'. He added reassuringly: 'I do not think your share in the theory will be overlooked by the real judges as Hooker, Lyell, [the American naturalist] Asa Gray &c. –'.[10]

No protestations about shared credit would shift the spotlight. The *Origin* was manifestly the product of an individual mind, however ably assisted. Hooker, whose help Darwin acknowledged fulsomely in the *Origin*, wrote on 21 November to thank Darwin 'for your glorious book – What a mass of close reasoning on curious facts & fresh phenomena – it is capitally written & will be very successful'. Characteristically for Hooker, there was no further engagement in the letter with that reasoning. Hooker had many virtues, scientific and personal; not for nothing had he become assistant director at the Royal Botanic Gardens at Kew and one of Darwin's closest confidantes. But he was not a thinker in anything like the same class as Lyell. Indeed, Hooker confessed that he had not even read the *Origin* through yet, having managed only '2 or 3 plunges into as many chapters'. But that was enough for him.[11] How different would be Huxley's response! Based at London's Royal School of Mines, Huxley was a thinker, indeed a brilliant one, with outsized intellectual appetites and powers of expression. Amid all the gossip in Hooker's letter, the item that cheered Darwin most was the news that Huxley – reported to be 'vastly pleased' with the book – was considering giving a Friday evening lecture on it in the prestigious series at London's Royal Institution, where the famous, and famously devout, natural philosopher Michael Faraday still presided. 'It would be unspeakably grand', Darwin wrote back, 'if Huxley were to lecture on the subject, but I can see this is mere chance: Faraday might think it too unorthodox'.[12]

Huxley in fact did manage to give his lecture, in early February 1860.[13] In the meantime, Darwin had Huxley's Ilkley-borne response to savour. Of all the letters Darwin received in Ilkley, Huxley's of 23 November is the one that mattered most in shaping the future of what, in only a few years' time, would come to be known as 'Darwinism'. It mattered first of all because Huxley here declared his devotion to the cause and his eagerness to serve. Huxley had written as soon as possible after finishing the book because, he explained, ever since his reading of the great German embryologist Karl Ernst von Baer's essays nine years before, 'no work on Natural History Science I have met with has made so great an impression upon me & I do most heartily thank you for the great store of new views you have given me'. For a large number of doctrines in the book, Huxley announced himself 'prepared to go to the Stake'. And he was in no doubt that vigorous defence would be needed. He wrote to Darwin:

> I trust you will not allow yourself to be in any way disgusted or annoyed by the considerable abuse
> & misrepresentation which unless I greatly mistake is in store for you – Depend upon it you have
> earned the lasting gratitude of all thoughtful men – And to the curs which will bark & yelp – you
> must recollect that some of your friends at any rate are endowed with an amount of combativeness
> which (though you have often & justly rebuked it) may stand you in good stead—

Never one to pass up the dramatic gesture, he added, 'I am sharpening up my claws & beak in readiness'.[14] He meant it: his savaging of Darwin's critics – above all the religiously motivated ones – would eventually earn Huxley the nickname 'Darwin's bulldog'. Anyone who today feels that Darwinism represents a bridge too far for traditional religion is the inheritor of Huxley's uncompromisingly polemical way of framing the issues on Darwinism's behalf.[15]

Yet the letter of the 23rd is equally important, and indeed is often quoted, for one of the criticisms that Huxley levelled at the *Origin*. Surely, Huxley suggested, 'you have loaded yourself with an unnecessary difficulty in adopting '*Natura non facit saltum*' [Nature makes no leaps] so unreservedly. I believe she does make small jumps'.[16] Darwin quoted that ancient maxim in the *Origin*; and it perfectly summed up his Lyellian conviction that all changes on the Earth and in its creatures came about slowly and smoothly, not quickly and jerkily.[17] For Huxley, however, those options were not mutually exclusive when it came to organisms. As he would later explain in his many public lectures and writings on Darwinian theory, continuous change at a low level of organisation – at, say, the level of the molecules making up the cells in the brain – could have cascading consequences which, at higher levels of organisation – the overall functionality of the brain itself – made for striking discontinuities. Such indeed, Huxley would suggest, accounted for the differences between the brains of apes, who could not speak, and the apparently very similar brains of humans, who could speak – an ability from which all else distinctively human flowed.[18] From the 1860s until his death in the 1890s, Huxley would remain a stubborn defender of the view that one could be both a Darwinian in good standing and someone who believed in natural leaps – a 'saltationist'. Throughout the twentieth century and even today, Darwinian saltationism has remained a minority view – never fully mainstream, but never completed eradicated either.[19]

Understandably, Darwin chose to dwell on the praise:

> Like a good Catholic, who has received extreme unction, I can now sing '*nunc dimittis*' [now you send
> forth (your servant, Lord) – a Biblical phrase]. I should have been more than contented with one

quarter of what you have said. Exactly fifteen months ago, when I put pen to paper for this volume, I had awful misgivings, & thought perhaps I had deluded myself like so many have done; & I then fixed in my mind three judges, on whose decision I determined mentally to abide. The judges were Lyell, Hooker & yourself. It was this which made me so excessively anxious for your verdict. I am now contented, & can sing my *nunc dimittis*. What a joke it will be if I pat you on back when you attack some immoveable creationist![20]

By this time, Lyell had confirmed by post what Hooker had been saying about him. Darwin's third judge – and the most important of all, his Lord High Chancellor – was now on-side, and prepared to say so publicly. Darwin was thrilled, and humbled. Nothing, Darwin ventured to Lyell in a letter of 23 November (Lyell's prompting letter has not been found), 'could be more important for [the theory's] success'. Darwin went on:

I honour you most sincerely: – to have maintained, in the position of a master, one side of a question for 30 years & then deliberately give it up, is a fact, to which I much doubt whether the records of science offer a parallel. For myself, also, I rejoice profoundly; for thinking of the many cases of men pursuing an illusion for years, often & often a cold shudder has run through me & I have asked myself whether I may not have devoted my life to a phantasy. Now I look at it as morally impossible that investigators of truth like you & Hooker can be wholly wrong; & therefore I feel that I may rest in peace.[21]

What of the other naturalists – 'the mob', as Darwin had rather disobligingly called them in one of his letters to Hooker? Darwin's other *Origin*-presaging letters from Ilkley went to some of the more distinguished representatives. English ones beyond Darwin's immediate circle form the third group of recipients; foreign men of science make up the fourth. Among those in the former group were two of his clerical Cambridge teachers, the botanist John Stevens Henslow and the geologist Adam Sedgwick. Darwin wrote to them both on 11 November. To Henslow, 'my dear old master in natural history', Darwin expressed concern that all the labour behind the book would not be visible, promising that he would start work on the 'bigger book' he had always intended shortly. Yet, though Henslow might well not approve of his former pupil, Darwin held out hope. He wrote that Henslow, on reading the book, would experience at least a slight wobble in his belief in the independent creation of species. Even a slight wobble would, Darwin reckoned, be victory, and no doubt the beginning of larger ones to follow; for, he continued (and as he had earlier written to Lyell), if 'you are in *ever so slight a degree* staggered (which I hardly expect) on the immutability of species, then I am convinced with further reflexion you will become more & more staggered, for this has been the process through which my mind has gone'.[22] The letter to Sedgwick was strikingly different – at once bolder and less optimistic. Darwin could well imagine, he wrote, that Sedgwick would see a 'spirit of bravado' and 'want of respect' behind a book that aimed to undermine a view of life which Sedgwick had long advocated. Yet, Darwin continued, 'I assure you that I am actuated by quite opposite feelings'.[23] That assurance would not, as we shall see, prove strong enough to pull Sedgwick to the cause. His letter of reply to Darwin would be the most hostile that he received in Ilkley.

Another teacher of sorts whose response to the *Origin* would ultimately disappoint was Sir John Herschel, whom Darwin wrote to on 11 November as well. Before embarking on

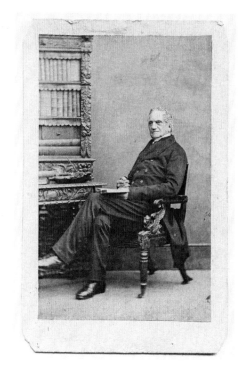

Reverend Adam Sedgwick (1785-1873). Yorkshire-born and Sedbergh-educated, Sedgwick was elected Professor of Geology at Cambridge University in 1818 and held the post for the rest of his life. (© National Portrait Gallery, London)

the *Beagle*, Darwin had read – and been transformed by – the astronomer Herschel's popular introductory book on scientific method, *A Preliminary Discourse on the Study of Natural Philosophy* (1830). Herschel was a friend and admirer of Lyell's, and held up his geology as the very model of good Newtonian reasoning about the causes of things. Later in the voyage, as the ship rounded South Africa, Darwin got to meet Herschel, and found him just as inspiring in person. Herschel was at that moment in soon-famous correspondence with Lyell over what Herschel called 'the mystery of mysteries': the replacement of old species by new.[24] Now, more than twenty years later, and with his life's work about to be published, Darwin was understandably moved as he contemplated Herschel and his role in it all. Darwin wrote to the older man that the book on species was being sent:

> ...with the hope that you may still retain some interest on this question... I cannot resist the temptation of showing in this feeble manner my respect, & the deep obligation, which I owe to your Introduction to Natural Philosophy. Scarcely anything in my life made so deep an impression on me: it made me wish to try to add my mite to the accumulated store of natural knowledge.[25]

Other English naturalists received less emotionally involved letters in advance of their copies arriving, among them the palaeontologist Hugh Falconer, the anatomist Richard Owen (who had sorted out Darwin's fossil finds from the *Beagle*), the naturalist Leonard Jenyns (who had done comparable work on the fish collected during the voyage), the geologist John Phillips, the botanist H.C. Watson, the physiologist William Carpenter, the farmer-naturalist Thomas Eyton, the banker-naturalist John Lubbock (a young neighbour in Kent) and the clergyman-naturalist

Charles Kingsley (whose 1863 children's classic *The Water Babies* has a strong Darwinian subtext). The letters were mostly variations on a stable set of themes: No doubt you will abhor my book! But do please read it through; and if, after reading it and thinking about it, you should find yourself ever so slightly doubtful about species immutability, well, just give yourself time; and as happened to me, and is now happening to such impeccable judges as Lyell and Hooker, you may well eventually concede the probable truth of my theory. For how could a theory that explains so much yet be false?[26]

'On these grounds I drop my anchor & believe that the difficulties will slowly disappear'.[27] So Darwin closed his letter to the Harvard botanist Asa Gray – one of several letters written to this same pattern and indeed on the same day, 11 November, that Darwin wrote to Henslow, Sedgwick and Herschel (as well as Falconer, Owen and Phillips). These other letters were headed overseas: to New England, where Gray's Harvard colleague Louis Agassiz would, like Gray, receive a copy of the *Origin*, as would the Yale geologist and zoologist James Dwight Dana; and to Switzerland, where the book would be entrusted to the botanist Alphonse de Candolle and the palaeontologist François Jules Pictet de la Rive.[28] As Darwin wrote to Carpenter, after receiving a positive reply, everything depended on bringing such figures aboard. 'If I am in the main right (of course including partial errors unseen by me) the admission of my views will depend far more on men, like yourself, with well established reputations, than on my own writings'.[29] Darwin would find out shortly what the world of established reputation had to say.

Notes

1   C.D. to J.D. Hooker, 15 October [1859]; Correspondence, 7, pp. 349–350, emphasis in original.

2   C.D. to T.H. Huxley, 15 October [1859]; Correspondence, 7, pp. 350–351, emphasis in original.

3   C.D. to John Murray, 15 October [1859]; Correspondence, 7, pp. 351–352.

4   John Murray to C.D., 2 November 1859 and C.D. to John Murray, [3 November 1859]; Correspondence, 7, pp. 364–365, emphasis in original. Although the letter to Murray is headed 'Wells Terrace' (i.e. North House), it is not clear that Darwin was there when he got his first look at the *Origin*, since Emma's diary records him returning to the house on 4 November from a temporary visit to the hotel; Correspondence, 7, p. 362, footnote 1.

5   Correspondence, 8, pp. 554–570; Browne, J., *Charles Darwin: The Power of Place* (Jonathan Cape, London 2002), pp. 86 and 507, footnote 13. Among the recipients was Mary Butler; Correspondance, 8, p. 559.

6   C.D. to W.D. Fox, [16 November 1859]; Correspondence, 7, pp. 377–378.

7   C.D. to Caroline Sarah Wedgwood, [after 21 November 1859]; Correspondence, 7, pp. 386–387. Darwin returned at much greater length to the origin(s) of domesticated dogs in the first chapter of his 1868 book *The Variation of Animals and Plants Under Domestication*.

8   Sloan, P., 'The making of a philosophical naturalist', in Hodge, J., and Radick, G. (eds), *The Cambridge Companion to Darwin*, 2nd edition (Cambridge University Press, Cambridge 2009), p. 23.

9   E.A. Darwin to C.D., 23 November [1859]; Correspondence, 7, p. 390.

10   C.D. to A.R. Wallace, 13 November 1859; Correspondence, 7, p. 375.

11   J.D. Hooker to C.D., [21 November 1859]; Correspondence, 7, p. 383. It was not just scientific merit that got Hooker his position at Kew; his father William was Kew's Director.

12 C.D. to J.D. Hooker, [22 November 1859]; Correspondence, 7, p. 387.

13 Correspondence, 7, footnote 4 (upper page). Titled 'On species and races, and their origin', Huxley's lecture can be read in summary (with some quotation) at http://math.clarku.edu/huxley/SM2/Sp-R.html

14 T.H. Huxley to C.D., 23 November 1859; Correspondence, 7, pp. 390–391.

15 On Huxley's role in promoting the idea that science and religion are incompatible – and, relatedly, that clergymen-naturalists have no place in professional science – see Turner, F., 'The Victorian conflict between science and religion: a professional dimension', *Isis*, 1978; 69: 356–376.

16 T.H. Huxley to C.D., 23 November 1859; Correspondence, 7, p. 391, emphasis in original. There was also another, less-famous objection that Huxley raised in this letter, concerning variation and the environment. '[I]t is not clear to me,' he wrote, 'why if external physical conditions are of so little moment as you suppose variation should occur at all'. (p. 391)

17 Darwin, C., *On the Origin of Species* (John Murray, London 1859), p. 471. Darwin invoked 'the canon of "*Natura non facit saltum*"' as capturing a truth that – once again – natural selection theory explains but the independent-creations theory cannot.

18 See, e.g., Huxley, T. H., *On Our Knowledge of the Causes of the Phenomena of Organic Nature* (Robert Hardwicke, London 1863), pp. 153–156.

19 A study that highlights Huxley's role in this alternative evolutionary tradition is Blitz, D., *Emergent Evolution: Qualitative Novelty and the Levels of Reality* (Kluwer, Dordrecht 1992).

20 C.D. to T.H. Huxley, 25 November [1859]; Correspondence, 7, p. 398.

21 C.D. to Charles Lyell, 23 November [1859]; Correspondence, 7, p. 392.

22 C.D. to J.S. Henslow, 11 November 1859; Correspondence, 7, p. 370, emphasis in original.

23 C.D. to Adam Sedgwick, 11 November 1859; Correspondence, 7, p. 373.

24 On the impact on Darwin of reading Herschel, see Sloan, P., 'The making of a philosophical naturalist', in Hodge, J., and Radick, G. (eds), *The Cambridge Companion to Darwin*, 2nd edition (Cambridge University Press, Cambridge 2009), pp. 27–28 and 39. On the impact of meeting Herschel, see Browne, J., *Charles Darwin: Voyaging* (Jonathan Cape, London 2002), pp. 328–330. Darwin quoted Herschel's phrase in the introduction to the *Origin*. Darwin, C., *On the Origin of Species* (John Murray, London 1859), p. 1 ('that mystery of mysteries, as it has been called by one of our greatest philosophers'). On Herschel's unimpressed reaction to the theory of natural selection ('the law of higgledy-piggledy' he called it), see Hull, D.H., 'Darwin's science and Victorian philosophy of science', in Hodge and Radick (2009), pp. 186-188.

25 C.D. to J.F.W. Herschel, 11 November [1859]; Correspondence, 7, pp. 370–371.

26 Letters to and/or from these men can be found in the Correspondence, 7, pp. 368–393.

27 C.D. to Asa Gray, 11 November [1859]; Correspondence, 7, p. 369.

28 Letters to these men can be found in the Correspondence, 7, pp. 366–372.

29 C.D. to W.B. Carpenter, 18 November [1859]; Correspondence, 7, p. 378.

Chapter Eight

Publication and Publicity

With Darwin's 'child' now imminent, his protective instincts came to the fore. In his letter to the physiologist Carpenter, Darwin warned that there would 'be strong opposition to my views'. It was all the more important, he continued, for the book's supporters to get their retaliation in first, above all through favourable reviews. Might Carpenter consider placing such a review himself, Darwin asked? True, Carpenter had so far read only the book's final, summarising chapter and it was not, Darwin acknowledged, an author's place to meddle in the review process. But meddle he did, expressing appreciation in advance for Carpenter's 'being willing to run the chance of unpopularity by advocating the view'. No doubt, Darwin added, a review from someone so accomplished would 'be excellently done & will do good service in the cause for which I think I am not selfishly, deeply interested'.[1] A follow-up note the next day from Darwin – perhaps remorseful about the presumptuousness of the letter – asked that Carpenter at least post something short, saying what he thought of the book. 'I could bear a hostile verdict', Darwin wrote, '& shall have to bear many a one'.[2]

That was on 19 November. With the book still five days from publication, the first review appeared in that day's issue of the *Athenaeum*, a popular London weekly. The anonymous reviewer – now known to be the coalfield commissioner and man of letters John Leifchild – was too ironical to count as hostile. He gently lampooned Darwin's parental concern for natural selection theory, noting how the *Origin*'s readers find the theory 'dandled like a loved infant of unquestioned paternity, and nourished with appropriate aliment':

> It grows fast as we turn over the pages, and by the time we have arrived at the last, it walks by itself, it gratifies its father by its sturdy progress, it brings smiles to his face so 'sicklied o'er with the pale cast of thought,' and you listen with wonder to the glorious future which he predicts for his hopeful progeny. Why for this rather than for other theories? Surely in obedience to the impulse of Natural Selection. It is most natural that a father should supremely love his own offspring, most natural that he should select it from all others as the favoured of the future, as the successful competitor in the struggle for existence.

Ribbing aside, the review gave an accurate and even-handed account of Darwin's major proposals and the range of evidence summoned to support them, from animal and plant breeding, palaeontology, the geographical distribution of species, classification and embryology. Leifchild noted how cleverly Darwin dealt with anticipated objections but also how unsatisfied his opponents, with good reason, might well remain. Without coming down on one side or the other, Leifchild raised the question of whether it was better theologically to suppose that God constantly intervenes in His creation, crafting each species independently, or to suppose instead, with Darwin, that God operates through natural law, for species-making as for everything else. On one point, however, Leifchild took a clear stand. '[N]either book, author, nor subject is of merely ordinary character,' he wrote. 'The work deserves attention, and will, we have no doubt, meet with it'.[3]

On 20 November, Darwin wrote to Hooker about the review. On the whole, Darwin thought it 'well done', though he was disappointed that the objections got so much attention, and confessed that he feared 'from tone of review that I have written in a conceited & cock-sure style, which shames me a little'.[4] By the next day, the review's criticisms loomed larger for him. He wrote to his sister Caroline, 'I have been cut up in *Athenaeum*, and under a theological point of view, unfairly'.[5] But then came cheering-up letters from his friends, full of praise for what they had read in their presentation copies. Now, he reckoned, he could take ungenerous reviews like this one in his stride. 'You have cockered me up to that extent, that I now feel I can face a score of savage Reviewers,' Darwin wrote to Hooker on 22 November.[6] And to John Lubbock that same day: 'I care not for Reviews, but for the opinion of men like you & Hooker & Huxley & Lyell &c'.[7]

It was, of course, Lyell's opinion that mattered most. For all that Lyell had been positive about the *Origin*, he had long withheld full assent, instead sending letter after letter of critical questioning. But, as we have seen, now even Lyell had been won over. On 23 November, Darwin wrote his letter thanking Lyell for his willingness to say so publicly, despite many years on the other side of the transmutation-of-species debate and also his reservations about Darwin's backing of a Pallasian story for the origins of domesticated dogs. Darwin in that letter assured Lyell that any religious backlash against the *Origin* would likely not affect him overmuch. Even 'if I am much execrated as atheist &c,' Darwin doubted that Lyell's 'admission of doctrine of natural Selection could injure [his] Works', since in general 'the virulence of bigotry is expended on first offender, & those who adopt his view are only pitied, as deluded, by the wise & cheerful bigots'.[8] (If Victorians had added smiley faces to their correspondence, Darwin would have added one here.)

And then came publication day, 24 November. When we learn now that the 1,100 copies of the *Origin* made available instantly sold out, exhausting the first print run, it is easy to imagine thronged bookshops up and down the land. In fact the shops never saw any copies. All were sold with minimal commotion two days earlier at John Murray's 'trade sale', when the book dealers and other backstage bulk buyers, such as Charles Edward Mudie, who ran a popular subscription lending library, placed their orders. Indeed, so successful was that sale, with 250 more orders than books (Mudie alone ordered 500), that Murray immediately wrote to Darwin with the news, and to suggest a second edition, to be published as soon as he could prepare it. Delighted that his loyal publisher would not now 'have cause to repent of publishing', Darwin wrote back on the 24th that he was happy to oblige with corrections for the new edition.[9] It would have to be a minimal affair, however, for as he explained that same day in a letter to Lyell, his Ilkley condition made anything more impossible. 'Now under water-cure with all nervous power directed to the skin, I cannot possibly do head-work, & I must make only actually necessary corrections'.[10]

No sooner had the work begun, however, than the post brought the unwelcome response of his old geology teacher, Sedgwick, to the first edition. 'I have read your book with more pain than pleasure,' wrote Sedgwick. 'Parts of it I admired greatly; parts I laughed at till my sides were almost sore; other parts I read with absolute sorrow; because I think them utterly false & grievously mischievous'. Throughout, on Sedgwick's reading, Darwin had presented assumption-based conclusions as if they were fact-based. Worse, he had done so in the cause of a theory that was not just false but wicked, in that, were it accepted as true, 'humanity in my mind, would suffer a damage that might brutalize it – & sink the human race into a lower grade of degradation than any into which it has fallen since its written records tell us of its history'. There were more than a few passages, Sedgwick continued, that 'greatly shocked my moral taste'. Nevertheless, he also insisted that none of this was personal, but rather sent 'in a spirit of brotherly love' from an 'old friend'.[11]

Darwin's reply of 26 November was monumentally restrained. He took it as a high compliment, he wrote, that Sedgwick felt the book worth disagreeing with so fully and frankly, though it grieved Darwin 'to have shocked a man whom I sincerely honour'. But no doubt, he went on, Sedgwick would not have wanted someone who had worked as long and hard as Darwin to hide his results. And now that they were in the public domain, their truth would be tested. Indeed,

ON

THE ORIGIN OF SPECIES

BY MEANS OF NATURAL SELECTION,

OR THE

PRESERVATION OF FAVOURED RACES IN THE STRUGGLE
FOR LIFE.

By CHARLES DARWIN, M.A.,
FELLOW OF THE ROYAL, GEOLOGICAL, LINNÆAN, ETC., SOCIETIES;
AUTHOR OF ' JOURNAL OF RESEARCHES DURING H. M. S. BEAGLE'S VOYAGE
ROUND THE WORLD.'

LONDON:
JOHN MURRAY, ALBEMARLE STREET.
1859.

The right of Translation is reserved.

Title page of the first edition of On the Origin of Species. As late as March 1859, Darwin had wanted the book's title to begin with the phrase An Abstract of an Essay, but Murray objected to the term 'abstract'.

wrote Darwin, 'there are so many workers that, if I be wrong I shall soon be annihilated; & surely you will agree that truth can be known only by rising victorious from every attack'. Darwin signed off insisting on his gratitude and continued friendship.[12] To his real friends, however, he was more dismissive. 'I have had a kind yet slashing letter against me from poor dear old Sedgwick, "who has laughed till his sides ached at my Book",' Darwin wrote to Huxley on 25 November.[13] A few days later Darwin sent Sedgwick's letter on to Lyell, with the comment: 'it is terribly muddled & really the first page seems almost childish'.[14] Lamenting in a subsequent letter his book's failure to stave off abuse of the sort that Sedgwick had meted out, Darwin confided to Lyell:

I fully believe that I owe the comfort of the next few years of my life to your generous support & that of a very few others: I do not think I am brave enough to have stood being odious without support. Now I feel as bold as a Lion. But there is one thing I can see I must learn, viz. to think less of myself & my book.[15]

With Murray awaiting the second edition however, and no family to distract him, the book remained Darwin's regular companion. The most famous change he made in preparing the new edition came in response to a letter of Lyell's of the 24th, warning Darwin off a conjecture in the sixth chapter as to how whales might evolve from bears. Suppose, Darwin ventured, that a race of bears in the habit of swimming around open-mouthed to catch insects – as the black bear in North America had been seen to do, hours on end, 'like a whale' – experienced no interruption in the insect supply and no competition from superior insect catchers, generation after generation. In that case natural selection would gradually sculpt the lineage descended from those bears into ever more efficient insect catchers, 'with larger and larger mouths, till a creature was produced as monstrous as a whale'.[16] Exactly what troubled Lyell about this scenario is not clear, since his letter has not been found. Lyell was himself fond of using imaginary examples to illustrate theoretical principles, so it is unlikely he took Darwin to task on this point. Be that as it may, Darwin wrote back that he would 'certainly leave out Whale & Bear'. In the event he kept them in the second edition, but hardly, retaining only a single sentence about the observed swimming bear, now described as 'almost like a whale'.[17]

Where Lyell prompted a cut, Charles Kingsley inspired an addition. In his letter of 18 November thanking Darwin for 'the unexpected honour of your book', Kingsley had indicated that in at least a couple of ways he was well-placed to read the book without prejudice. First of all, he had come, through his own observations of domesticated plants and animals, to doubt the immutability of species. Second, he now saw 'that it is just as noble a conception of Deity, to believe that he created primal forms capable of self development... as to believe that He required a fresh act of intervention to supply the lacunas wh[ich] he himself had made'.[18] Impressed with Kingsley's way of putting the latter view, Darwin asked permission to quote from the letter. A lightly polished version, attributed to a 'celebrated author and divine', duly appeared in the second edition.[19]

By 2 December, Darwin had completed the work on the new edition. 'I have made some few corrections,' Darwin wrote to Murray that day, '& have inserted capital sentence from Rev C. Kingsley in answer to anyone who may, as many will, say that my Book is irreligious'. Even so, Darwin reckoned that the book would receive unfavourable reviews.[20] The next day's issue of the *Examiner* bore him out. The reviewer, an Orientalist named John Crawfurd, had sent word to Darwin beforehand about what to expect, as Darwin recounted to Lyell (Crawfurd's letter has not been found). 'Crawfurd writes to me that his notice will be hostile, but that "he will not calumniate the author"'.[21] Indeed Crawfurd was respectfully unpersuaded. For him, there was no doubting Darwin's remarkable talents as an investigator and author, or that these were on display throughout the *Origin*. Yet the problems with the new argument seemed to him insurmountable. Variation in nature was rare and usually debilitating. There was, among the human races as throughout nature, 'a natural repugnance to intermixture' that told against anything like Darwin's theory. Where Darwin envisaged progress, the rocks testified to occasional degeneration, with the replacement of more powerful species (mastodons, dinosaurs) by less powerful ones (elephants, crocodiles). In extending this last point Crawfurd drew perceptively on his knowledge of Eastern religions:

> The theory... is a scientific metempsychosis, not only more ingenious but far more consolatory than that of Hindus and Buddhists, for it is all hopeful progress without any counterbalance of melancholy retrogression, or still worse, of annihilation.[22]

Fortunately, the favourable notices had started to come as well. Among the first was one by Huxley, in the December issue of *Macmillan's Magazine*. It was not a review – Huxley would write one of those for *The Times* later in the month – but an analysis of recent discussions on the history of life and the history of the Earth with, as a kind of appendix, a lucid account of the theory of natural selection. Huxley explained that this unusual, two-part structure was appropriate because his conclusions in the first part – about transmutation as the only origin-of-species hypothesis with any scientific potential, and one which, when used to interpret the evidence of long-stable types of animals and plants in the fossil record, supports the view that the Earth is extremely old – had been much influenced by his acquaintance over recent years with Darwin. Now that Darwin had gone public with his own version of the transmutation hypothesis, it was timely to explore that version and the evidence in its favour. 'And I do this the more willingly,' Huxley added, 'as I observe that already the hastier sort of critics have begun, not to review my friend's book, but to howl over it in a manner which must tend greatly to distract the public mind'.

There followed a summary of Darwin's case in the first four chapters of the *Origin* for natural selection, concentrating on how, through selection for useful variations, breeders generate new varieties among domesticated plants and animals, and how, thanks to the struggle for existence, that 'which takes the place of the breeder and selector in nature is Death'. Huxley did not endorse natural selection theory, so much as welcome its testing:

> If it can be proved that the process of natural selection, operating upon any species, can give rise to varieties of species so different from one another that none of our tests will distinguish them from true species, Mr. Darwin's hypothesis of the origin of species will take its place among the established theories of science, be its consequences whatever they may. If, on the other hand, Mr. Darwin has erred, either in fact or in reasoning, his fellow-workers will soon find out the weak points in his doctrines, and their extinction by some nearer approximation to the truth will exemplify his own principle of natural selection... It is the duty of the general public to await the result in patience; and, above all things, to discourage, as they would any other crimes, the attempt to enlist the prejudices of the ignorant, or the uncharitableness of the bigoted, on either side of the controversy.[23]

On seeing the review, Darwin wrote to say how delighted he was with it while managing nevertheless to register his disappointment that Huxley had ignored most of the book. For Darwin, the important test of the theory was not the one that Huxley proposed but rather the theory's power to explain so many diverse bodies of biological fact, in palaeontology, biogeography and so on. 'It seems to me,' Darwin wrote to Huxley on 5 December, 'that the turning point on the reception of theory of N. selection will be whether or not it explains the recognised laws' in these areas. 'Those, like Crawfurd in *Examiner*, who have never troubled themselves on such points will reject it'.[24]

By now, however, Darwin had learned that his wooing of Carpenter had worked; he was writing a review for the *National Review*. 'It is a great thing to have got a great physiologist on our side', Darwin wrote to Carpenter on 3 December. 'I say "our" for we are now a good & compact body of really good men & mostly not old men.— In the long run we shall conquer'.[25] Darwin kept up this them-or-us talk in a letter to Lyell that day, crowing about the new convert and wondering about a review from Richard Owen. 'How curious I shall be to know what line Owen will take, – dead against us I fear; but he wrote me a *most* liberal note on the reception of my Book, & said he was quite prepared to consider fairly, & without prejudice any line of argument'.[26]

In English science and letters, then, the *Origin* was making its presence felt. But what of the world beyond? One of Darwin's final surviving letters from Ilkley, sent to the French palaeontologist Quatrefages on 5 December, dealt at length with the matter of a French translation. Quatrefages had responded positively to the copy of the *Origin* that Darwin had sent him; now Darwin brought him up to date on developments. Lyell, Hooker, Carpenter and Huxley had all been converted, as had other naturalists, and were preparing to say so publicly. The first edition had sold out on the first day, and the publisher was now printing 3,000 copies of a new edition. Meanwhile, a woman named Louise Belloc, an Irish-born translator of

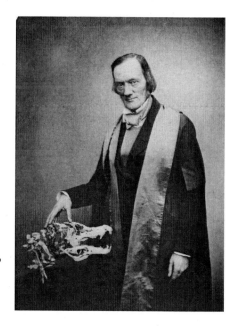

Richard Owen (1804-92). Born in Lancaster and based, from 1856, at the British Museum, Owen – who coined the term 'dinosauria' – was the leading British comparative anatomist of his generation.
(© National Portrait Gallery, London)

English books into French, had been in touch to ask about translating the *Origin*, having heard about it from friends. But now, Darwin reported, Madame Belloc had seen the book, and felt herself too unscientific to do it justice. However, their exchange had emboldened Darwin, as he explained to Quatrefages (from whom he was about to ask a favour), to think even bigger about the book. 'Now this has put it into my head,' wrote Darwin, 'what an immense advantage it would be, if it were translated. It would then be known to the world. I wish for this far more, (if I know myself) for the sake of the subject, than for my own reputation'.[27]

Notes

1   C.D. to W.B. Carpenter, 18 November [1859]; Correspondence, 7, pp. 378–379.

2   C.D. to W.B. Carpenter, 19 November [1859]; Correspondence, 7, p. 381.

3   [Leifchild, J.R.], review of the *Origin, Athenaeum*, 19 November 1859: 659–660. The quotation is from Hamlet's 'to be or not to be' soliloquy.

4   C.D. to J.D. Hooker, [20 November 1859]; Correspondence, 7, p. 382.

5   C.D. to C.S. Wedgwood, [after 21 November 1859]; Correspondence, 7, p. 386.

6   C.D. to J.D. Hooker, [22 November 1859]; Correspondence, 7, p. 387.

7   C.D. to John Lubbock, [22 November 1859]; Correspondence, 7, p. 388.

8   C.D. to Charles Lyell, 23 November [1859]; Correspondence, 7, p. 392.

9   C.D. to John Murray, 24 November [1859]; Correspondence, 7, p. 395. On the sale, see Correspondence, 7, footnote 1, p. 394 and footnote 1, p. 395.

10   C.D. to Charles Lyell, 24 [November 1859]; Correspondence, 7, p. 394.

11   Adam Sedgwick to C.D., 24 November 1859; Correspondence, 7, pp. 396–398.

12   C.D. to Adam Sedgwick, 26 November [1859]; Correspondence, 7, pp. 403–404.

13   C.D. to T.H. Huxley, 25 November [1859]; Correspondence, 7, p. 399.

14   C.D. to Charles Lyell, 29 [November 1859]; Correspondence, 7, p. 406.

15   C.D. to Charles Lyell, 2 December [1859]; Correspondence, 7, p. 409.

16   Darwin, C., *On the Origin of Species* (John Murray, London 1859), p. 184.

17   C.D. to Charles Lyell, 25 [November 1859]; Correspondence, 7, p. 400. See footnote 2 for the change made for the second edition, published on 7 January 1860.

18   Charles Kingsley to C.D., 18 November 1859; Correspondence, 7, pp. 379–380.

19   C.D. to Charles Kingsley, 30 November [1859]; Correspondence, 7, p. 407. See footnote 4 on p. 380 for the version and attribution in the second edition.

20   C.D. to John Murray, 2 December [1859]; Correspondence, 7, pp. 410–411.

21   C.D. to Charles Lyell, 2 December [1859]; Correspondence, 7, p. 409.

22   [Crawfurd, J], review of the *Origin, Examiner*, 3 December 1859: 772–773.

23   Huxley, T.H., 'Time and life: Mr. Darwin's "Origin of Species"', *Macmillan's Magazine*, December 1859; 1: 142–148, quotations on pp. 146–148.

24   C.D. to T.H. Huxley, [5 December 1859]; Correspondence, 7, p. 415.

25   C.D. to W.B. Carpenter, 3 December [1859]; Correspondence, 7, p. 412.

26   C.D. to Charles Lyell, [3 December 1859]; Correspondence, 7, p. 413, emphasis in original. For Owen's letter, see Richard Owen to C.D., 12 November 1859; Correspondence, 7, pp. 373–374.

27   C.D. to J.L.A. Quatrefages de Bréau, 5 December [1859]; Correspondence, 7, p. 416.

Chapter Nine

A Medical Postscript

Once the date of publication had passed, Darwin's health took a turn for the better. On 30 November he wrote to Charles Kingsley in a more positive frame of mind. 'I shall stay here at furthest only seven or eight days... during great part of day I am wandering on the hills, & trying to inhale health'.[1] Two weeks after being unable to walk because of swollen legs and a 'boil' on his knee, Darwin was wandering the hills – a remarkable recovery. Could it have been directly linked with the long-awaited appearance in print of his 'abominable' book?

Darwin left Wells House on 7 December and journeyed to London where he stayed with his brother, Erasmus. He used the short stay in London as an opportunity to visit Charles Lyell to discuss amendments for the second edition of the book, which they did over a late breakfast on Thursday 8th.[2] The next day Darwin travelled from London to Down House, there to be reunited with his beloved Emma, the children, his study and his Sand Walk. Over the next few weeks, Darwin's letters reveal an all-too-short benefit from his nine weeks of water cure. On 14 December, he declared: 'The latter part of my stay at Ilkley did me much good; but I suppose I never shall be strong, for the work I have had since I came back has knocked me up a little more than once'.[3] By the 21st, his poor health was once again interfering with his work. 'I will write again in a few days,' he told Asa Gray, 'for I am at present unwell & much pressed with business'.[4] On the same day, he wrote to Hooker, 'I had hoped to come up for the Club tomorrow, but very much doubt whether I shall be able. Ilkley seems to have done me no essential good'.[5] Two days later, he qualified this negative conclusion. 'Ilkley did me extraordinary good during the latter part of my stay & during my first week at home; but I have gone back latterly to my bad way & fear I shall never be decently well and strong'.[6] He repeated this analysis in a letter written on Christmas Day:

> The last 10 days at Ilkley, I was splendidly well & for the first week at home; but since then I have had as bad a week as man could well have with incessant discomfort, I may say misery. – I have necessarily been very busy during these weeks but not with work which would be any strain to any other mortal man. I was hardly able through lameness, Boils &c to give Water-cure a fair trial this time, but I think we shall go there again early next summer.[7]

The progress of Darwin's illness during his autumn stay in Ilkley and over the ensuing few weeks is important for our understanding of the nature of his condition. He arrived at Wells House

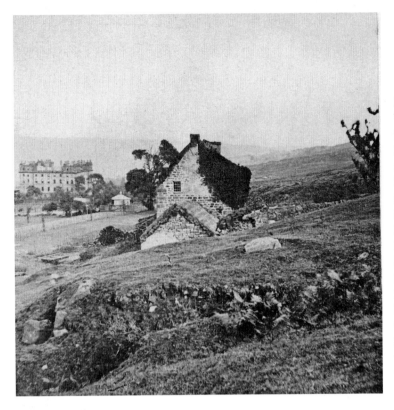

Hill Top Farm with Wells House in the background. Darwin occupied the last ten days in Ilkley 'wandering on the hills, & trying to inhale health'. Inevitably, one of his walks would have been up the Keighley (Gate) Road that would have given him this view back to the hotel. The cottage was demolished in the 1890s. (Gordon Burton)

on 4 October complaining of recurrent vomiting, fatigue and weakness – problems that he had endured with varying severity for many years. After just ten days treatment, he was able to state that the water cure had done him much good. On the 17th he moved out of Wells House to join his family in North House. Six days later he complained of an eruption and inflammation of the legs brought about by the wet-bandages, but felt his stomach to be 'wonderfully good'. Later he complained of swelling of the face and legs, and a rash with boils (the latter may be directly attributable to the water treatment). After six weeks' treatment, Darwin claimed to feel worse than when he arrived and had difficulty walking. On 24 November his family left for the South and he moved back into Wells House, whereupon his condition improved. During the last ten days in Ilkley, Darwin was so reinvigorated that he was able to take walks on the moor.

The improvement cannot be explained by a period of rest and relaxation following the publication date. From the day of publication, Darwin was, as we have seen, engaged on amendments for a second edition that John Murray had demanded instantly. An important negative observation is that at no time during his stay did his letters make mention of vomiting. But the positive health note on which he left Ilkley rapidly faded. After only a week at home, he became unwell and in the following week complained of 'incessant discomfort'. The nature of the discomfort was not made explicit so we cannot confirm when flatulence and vomiting returned, but return they did.

Looking at this medical narrative in isolation, one could summarise it as follows: Darwin was ill when he arrived at Wells House; he got better while he was in the hotel; became ill

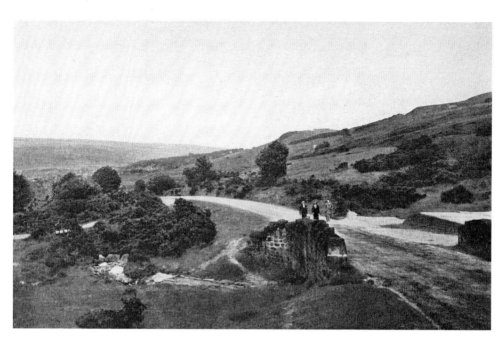

Higher up, Keighley Road crosses Spicey Gill. From this point, the walker has wonderful views over mid-Wharfedale. The road then climbs to the top of the moor from where there are views into Airedale.

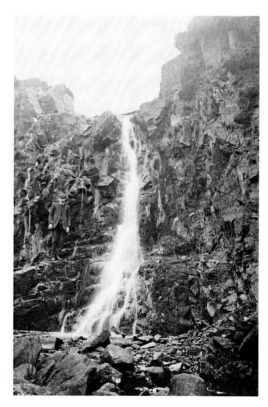

Wandering over Ilkley Moor, Darwin could have visited Backstone Beck waterfall…

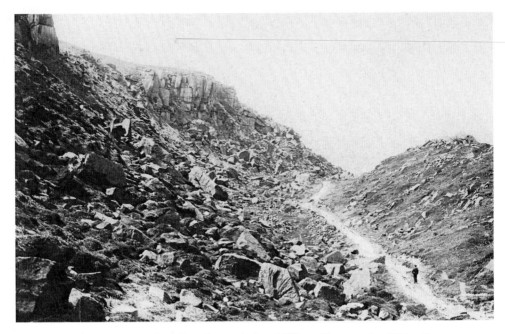

...and the rugged grandeur of Rocky Valley, with the cliff-like millstone grit of Ilkley Crags towering above.

with swollen legs and skin problems when he left the hotel and was reunited with his family; got better when he returned to the hotel; and relapsed when he got back home. In this much-abbreviated form, we could conclude that as far as Darwin's health is concerned, it was a matter of hotel good/home care bad. It will be important to bear this pattern in mind when considering the cause of his illness.

Although Darwin proposed a return visit to Ilkley, it did not happen. Nevertheless, his experiences at Wells House did not destroy his faith in the water cure. In his final letter of 1859, Darwin advocated hydropathy to his American correspondent Dana, who had recently suffered a breakdown.[8] Interestingly, Darwin's letter begins with an invocation for help from a deity whose existence he had privately repudiated. 'My dear Mr. Dana, I am most truly & deeply grieved at the news in your letter. God grant that you may soon recover'. Darwin went on to attest to the power of water treatment:

> Most regular medical men sneer at the Water-cure (I do not at all know whether it is adopted in the U. States)[9] but I have tried it repeatedly & always with wonderfully good effects, but not permanent in my case. When I first tried it, I could not sleep & whatever I did in the day haunted me at night with vivid & most wearing repetition. The W. cure at once relieved this. It makes the skin act so vigorously that all other organs get a rest. For years I have been in your state, that an hour's conversation worked me up to that degree that I wished myself dead. But then my head never ultimately suffers; for my peccant part is the stomach & fatigue of any kind always brings on great derangement & ultimately severe vomiting. So that the weak organ seems to save the more important one.

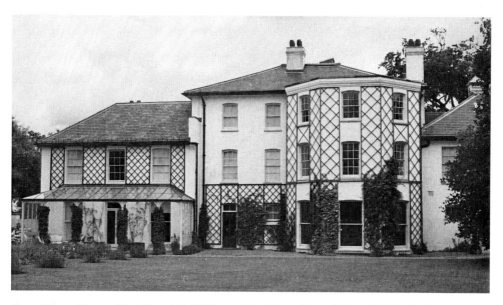

Down House, Downe, Kent. Darwin left Ilkley on the 7 December and arrived back at his home on the 9th after two nights with his brother Erasmus in London. His return home signalled yet another deterioration in his health, reversing the improvement he experienced in his last ten days at the hotel in Ilkley. (Sandra Hanby)

Darwin was to resort to the water cure on at least two further occasions. In June 1860, with his stomach 'utterly broken down' he felt forced to go for a week's water cure at Dr Edward Lane's new establishment at Sudbrook Park in Richmond, Surrey.[10] Then in 1863, suffering 'a bad amount of sickness', he overcame his fears over a return to Malvern and placed himself under Dr James Smith Ayerst at the Old Well House in Malvern Wells.[11] After four weeks' treatment, Darwin wrote: 'I am very weak & can write little. – My nervous system has failed & I am kept going only by repeated doses of brandy; but I am certainly better, much, & sickness stopped'.[12] He stayed at Malvern for eight weeks but, once again, the relief from vomiting was short-lived. Two weeks after his return to Down, Darwin's local doctor, Dr Engleheart, went up to London to consult a leading specialist in stomach disorders, Dr William Brinton, on Darwin's behalf. He brought back a prescription, and Brinton himself visited Darwin at Down House in November and December 1863, but the specialist's ministrations provided no lasting benefit.[13]

After 1863, Darwin abandoned the water cure and became a martyr to flatulence and almost daily vomiting. There followed long periods when he felt unable to work such was his discomfort and weakness. He continued to try novel treatments, including the bizarre approach of applying ice-bags to the spine, and occasionally enjoyed some respite – only to relapse a short time later. In subsequent years he staggered from relapse to remission in a repeated cycle, dogged by vomiting and fatigue, working during the better periods and suffering enforced idleness at other times.

In the last decade of his life (1872-82), Darwin lived the life of the authentic 'invalid recluse', a role in which he had long been cast, but not always with justification. Surprisingly for someone with a chronic illness, his general health underwent a significant improvement during these final years. Without the distraction of caring for children, Emma was able to devote all her attention to her husband's well-being, and he appeared to respond. In his last few years his letters reveal few complaints, and because of the improvement in his stomach condition, he was able to work more steadily.[14] Only in his last few months of life did serious illness return. Towards the end of 1881, he complained of giddiness and an irregular pulse, and developed chest pain in March 1882, which was diagnosed as angina. The pain became more persistent and severe. His condition gradually deteriorated and he died following a heart attack on 19 April 1882.

From a medical point of view, the cause of death is the only aspect of Darwin's illness on which there is unanimity. Certainly there was no firm diagnosis in life. Darwin exhibited a multitude of symptoms, but despite consulting some of the finest physicians in the land, not one came up with a single physical finding of diagnostic usefulness. Thus, all was speculation during Darwin's lifetime, and the conjecture has continued ever since. We cannot go into all the possibilities. Every biomedical scientist who has looked into Darwin's medical history can find some support for his or her own individual theory, and this has led to a plethora of diagnoses. The following three categories represent the main possibilities.

1. Darwin had a mental disorder

The first psychiatric diagnosis attached to Darwin's illness was hypochondriasis – a state of chronic anxiety about imagined health problems. Indeed, some of Darwin's friends considered him to be a hypochondriac. A modern interpretation might be that he had a form of somatisation disorder, in which the patient complains of multiple, recurrent physical symptoms in the absence of any underlying 'organic' medical explanation.[15] Symptoms may be referred to any part or system of the body, but gastrointestinal sensations (pain, belching, regurgitation, vomiting, nausea, etc.), and abnormal skin sensations (itching, burning, tingling, numbness, soreness, etc.) and blotchiness are among the commonest. Thus, the similarity between a somatisation disorder and Darwin's illness is clear to see. A key feature of this diagnosis, however, is that the symptoms are frequently changing. Although Darwin had a multiplicity of symptoms, they were remarkably consistent in their pattern.

Over the years, numerous psychiatrists have concluded that Darwin suffered from a psychoneurosis, brought on by emotional turmoil.[16] But the conflicts so far identified as possibly bringing about this turmoil have often been exaggerated or downright spurious. Some writers have invoked conflict with an over-bearing father. Others have cited anxiety over the consequences for religious belief of his transmutation theory, and in particular over the effect on Emma – a woman with a strong Christian faith. Yet others have blamed anxiety over the hostile reception his book would receive among the scientific community. Such explanations, together with some (for twenty-first-century tastes) far-fetched Freudian variations, can never be dismissed altogether. But neither, it seems, can their loose ties with the evidence be made any tighter. The range of physical symptoms he displayed is very difficult to reconcile with a purely psychiatric diagnosis, even if one allows for the role of stress in many of these complaints.

For this reason, some authors have suggested that Darwin's problems were psychosomatic, combining mind and body, and that his psychoneurosis overlay an 'organic' disease affecting the digestive system – though quite what the underlying disease is has typically been left vague.[18] Similarly, given Darwin's complex pattern of symptoms, candidate diagnoses such as panic disorder with agoraphobia[19] and bipolar disorder[20] appear untenable as the main cause of his illness. Both could also be refuted on the grounds of their principal psychiatric features and plausibility.

Whatever the psychiatric or psychosomatic diagnosis favoured, a related argument has long had it that Darwin's symptoms, and his excessive anxiety over them, functioned to erect a protective barrier that facilitated study and writing, helping Darwin to avoid the social and academic commitments that would distract him from his life's work.[17] The hollowness of this view is plain to see, as Darwin made numerous references to illness and indisposition that prevented him from working, and to his frustration over the time he lost on his various projects.

2. Darwin had Chagas' disease (South American trypanosomiasis)

The proposition that while in South America Darwin contracted an exotic infection that led to a chronic, debilitating illness is an attractive one. It combines a permanent, if unfortunate, legacy of his *Beagle* adventure with the desire by many to find an organic explanation for his illness. As such, the suggestion that Darwin was suffering from Chagas' disease – first put forward in 1959[21] – met with enthusiastic acceptance by several commentators.[22]

Chagas' disease was not a diagnosis available to Darwin's doctors. It was discovered by, and named after, Dr Carlos Chagas, who recognised the infection while working in the Amazon basin in 1908-9. The disease is a protozoan parasitic infection, trypanosomiasis, spread through the bite of an insect vector, the vinchuca bug (Darwin called it a 'Benchuca'). The blood-sucking vinchucas (*Triatoma infestans*) transmit the pathogenic trypanosomes (*Trypanosoma cruzi*) to man when the bug's infected faeces contaminate their bites, as happens for instance if the bug is crushed at the moment of biting. Once the trypanosomes have entered through the skin, they multiply locally and are then carried through the blood stream to infect muscle tissue at distant sites, including the heart muscle.[23]

There is no doubting that Darwin was bitten by this bug while on an inland trek in Mendoza Province in Argentina on 25 March 1835, for he records in his *Beagle* diary that he 'experienced an attack (for it deserves no less a name) of the Benchuca, a species of Reduvius, the great black bug of the Pampas'.[24] Not all vinchucas carry the infection, however, and transmission is not inevitable. Darwin reported no painful nodule or sore at the site of a bite which, although not an invariable feature, is characteristic of the acute phase of infection. The chronic phase begins about two months after infection; but over the remaining eighteen months of the voyage, Darwin exhibited robust good health. More tellingly, the chronic features of Chagas' disease do not accord with Darwin's symptoms. The persistent infection, and the body's immunological reaction to it, principally involves the heart and the upper digestive tract. [23] Thus, the classical features are damage to heart muscle producing heart failure, and involvement of the intrinsic nerves of the oesophagus (gullet) and colon, giving rise to difficulties with swallowing, regurgitation of food, vomiting and constipation.

After examining the features of Darwin's illness and other relevant data, one expert in tropical medicine pointed out several discrepancies with the diagnosis of Chagas' disease, namely:

> Darwin's good exercise tolerance, the absence of physical signs of organic disease, the absence of evidence of Chagas' disease among the other members of the *Beagle* crew, the fact that the illness was compatible with long life although Darwin suffered from it for more than 50 years [actually it was 47 years], and the fact that his symptoms improved towards the end of his life. Each of these would cause doubts, and some of them grave doubts, about a diagnosis of Chagas' disease, but taken collectively they make a case of overwhelming strength against it.[25]

3. Darwin had lactose intolerance (sensitivity)

The rejection of Chagas' disease as a cause of Darwin's illness leaves the field open for other non-psychiatric diagnoses.[26] Recently, the diagnosis of lactose intolerance (sensitivity) has been proposed, and this comes closest to accounting for all his symptoms and has a good deal of circumstantial evidence to support it.[27]

Before we look at the match between Darwin's complaints and the symptoms of lactose intolerance, it will help to consider the scientific basis of this condition. Lactose is a sugar found in milk and dairy products. Formed from two simpler sugars, glucose and galactose, lactose cannot be digested by the body until it is broken into these constituents by an enzyme called lactase which is secreted by, and present on, the cells lining the human small intestine. If lactase does not split lactose molecules as they pass through the small intestine, then not only is the body deprived of sugar (a source of energy) but, on reaching the large intestine, the intact lactose then undergoes gas-producing fermentation by colonic bacteria. The result is the formation of hydrogen and methane gas and toxic breakdown products that can have clinical consequences.

Fittingly, scientists can now supplement this biochemical story with a Darwinian one. Although humans have always produced lactase at birth in order to utilise the lactose in maternal milk, lactase production in our ancestors 'switched off' after only a few months, i.e. about the normal time of weaning. Between six and ten thousand years ago, however, a change in lactase production came about in communities that moved towards an agrarian economy. With cows and goats now increasing the milk supply, there was a survival advantage to being able to consume milk. For one thing, there was less risk of fatal diarrhoeal diseases compared to drinking water from potentially contaminated supplies. For another, milk drinking maintained a supply of valuable nutrients to children when other foodstuffs became scarce. Against this background, some individuals who had acquired a mutation in the gene that switched off lactase production were able to consume milk without ill-effects throughout their lifetime.[28] Lactase production therefore came under the influence of natural selection, and over the millennia, the genetic mutations that rendered people permanent lactase producers became widespread in milk-drinking populations. In northern Europeans, North Americans and Australasians, up to 95 per cent of adults are 'lactase persistent'; whereas in South America, Africa and Asia, rates range from fifty down to zero. Individuals who have the 'ancestral type' gene that switches off lactase production are at risk of the effects of lactose intolerance if they continue to consume milk and dairy products into adult life. Whether or not they develop symptoms will depend on the amount of lactose in their diet and the overall deficiency of lactase production (generally it has to be below 50 per cent of normal activity).[29] It can take eighteen to twenty years for lactase production to fall to below this threshold and give rise to clinical effects.[30]

The symptoms of lactose intolerance are shown in Table 1. Interestingly, in addition to the expected gut-related symptoms there are several generalised (systemic) effects due to the absorption of toxic metabolites from the large intestine. The table also shows the symptoms that Darwin exhibited, except for the dubious ones of 'depression' and 'anxiety' or feelings of panic. As to the former, there is no convincing evidence that he suffered from true depression as opposed to episodes of dejection or 'low mood'.[17] Such dejection, and occasional loss of control manifested by anxiety and panic attacks, could be expected in someone who had suffered from an undiagnosed, debilitating chronic disease for forty years and who was accused of imagining his symptoms.[27]

Digestive system symptom	% of patients with the symptom	Darwin	Systemic symptom	% of patients with the symptom	Darwin
Flatulence (gas in the digestive tract)	100	Yes	Headaches or light-headedness	86	Yes
Abdominal distension	100	Yes	Loss of concentration and poor short-term memory	82	Yes
Excessive bowel sounds	100	?	Long-term severe tiredness	63	Yes
Abdominal pain	100	Yes	Muscle pain	71	Yes
Nausea	78	Yes	Joint pain, and/or swelling and stiffness	40	Yes
Vomiting	78	Yes	Allergy (eczema, hay fever, rhinitis, sinusitis)	40	Yes
Diarrhoea	70	No	Mouth ulcers	30	Yes
Constipation	30	Yes	Palpitations and rhythm disturbances	24	Yes

Table 1: Symptoms exhibited by patients with lactose intolerance compared with the features of Darwin's illness (modified from 27 and 31)

While the overlap between the symptoms exhibited by Darwin and those seen in patients with lactose intolerance is striking, we should also emphasise that in the individual patient the pattern of symptoms will be influenced by other factors such as their state of mind (anxiety, self-preoccupation, childhood stress, bereavement), by their threshold level for discomfort in the intestine, and by reflex brain-gut interactions. Subjects with lactose intolerance (like some people with irritable bowel syndrome[32]) have been shown to be more aware of abdominal discomfort than normal subjects.[33] In Darwin's case, the brain-gut axis was especially relevant. Five years of almost daily sea-sickness on the *Beagle* voyage could have 'conditioned' Darwin to over-react to visceral sensations by reflex vomiting.[34] Because of such conditioning, Darwin might have responded to low-intensity visceral stimuli by vomiting, when in another individual the same sensations would have passed unnoticed, or at most led to a feeling of nausea. Darwin himself seems to have been peculiarly aware of brain-gut interactions. 'I find the noddle & stomach are antagonistic powers,' he explained to his sister, Caroline, 'and that it is a great deal more easy to think too much in a day, than to think too little – What this has to do with digesting roast beef, – I cannot say, but they are brother faculties'.[35] Later, he confessed to Hooker that he had worked the brain too much at the expense of the stomach.[36]

That the intestine and not the stomach was the source of the triggering sensations leading to Darwin's vomiting is in keeping with its delayed onset. 'You ask about my sickness – it rarely comes on till 2-3 hours after eating, so that I seldom throw up food, only acid & morbid secretion; otherwise I shd. have been dead, for during more than a month I vomited after every meal & several times most nights'.[37] The relationship between the intestine, stomach and brain in the genesis of Darwin's illness is nowhere better exemplified than in some notes that he and Emma drew up prior to a consultation with a Dr John Chapman. They wrote:

> Age 56-57.- For 25 years extreme spasmodic daily & nightly flatulence: occasional vomiting, on two occasions prolonged during months. Vomiting preceded by shivering, hysterical crying, dying sensations or half-faint, & copious very pallid urine. Now vomiting and every paroxys[m] of flatulence preceded by singing of ears, rocking, treading on air & vision… Tongue crimson in morning ulcerated – stomach constricting dragging… Appetite good – not thin. Evacuation regular & good. – Seldom headache or nausea – Cannot walk abv ½ mile – always tired – conversation or excitement tires me much… Eczema – (now constant) lumbago – fundament – rash… I fancy that when much sickness my stomach is cold – at least water is very little warmed. I feel nearly sure that the air is generated some where lower down than the stomach & as soon as it regurgitates into the stomach the discomfort comes on – Does not throw up the food.[38]

This short account is remarkable for the consistency between the digestive and systemic features that Darwin described and the actual symptoms of lactose intolerance. It is noteworthy that the first complaint he mentions is of 'extreme spasmodic daily & nightly flatulence'. Flatulence, the generation of gas in the digestive tract, is a cardinal feature of lactose intolerance.

Given Victorian sensitivities, it is perhaps understandable that the subject of flatulence was not explicitly described by Darwin as 'breaking wind' or the passage of *flatus* (from the Latin 'blowing'). In consequence, the symptom is open to some ambiguity. Colp, for example, tends to interpret Darwin's flatulence as eructation, i.e. originating in the stomach, and associated with vomiting,[39] but there is substantial evidence that it was largely an intestinal problem. As in the account of his symptoms above, Darwin concludes that the gas is generated 'lower down than the stomach', and there are several occasions where the distinction between his vomiting and 'fits' of flatulence is made clear.[40] After his first course of hydropathy at Malvern, he wrote, 'I consider the sickness is absolutely cured. And about 3 weeks since, I had 12 hours without any flatulence, which showed me that it was possible that even that can be cured, as Dr G. [Gully] has always said he could'.[41] There are times when Darwin appears to be more discomforted by flatulence than any other symptom, as when he wrote, 'All excitement & fatigue brings on such dreadful flatulence; that in fact I can go nowhere'.[42] In January 1866, he reported back to Dr Bence Jones, a leading London physician, on the effect of a new treatment regime. 'The only drawback is that on most days 3 hours after luncheon or dinner, I have a sharpish headache on one side, & with bad flatulence lasting to the next meal'.[43] In a subsequent reply from Bence Jones, the physician recommended that Darwin should 'get a rough pony & be shaken once daily to make the chemistry go on better'.[44] This advice had little to do with 'chemistry'. Dr Bence Jones would have been well aware that Darwin was much more likely to 'break wind' while jogging around on a horse in the fresh air than he would in the confines of his house, and that this would greatly benefit his abdominal discomfort. Accepting this advice,

Darwin bought a steady old gelding called Tommy from a local dealer, and for a year or two went on daily rides along the country paths before taking a bad tumble and deciding he was too old for the venture.[45] No doubt he went back to striding around the Sand Walk to achieve the same objective.

If we are to attribute Darwin's illness to lactose intolerance, one aspect of his lifestyle is of fundamental importance, namely the content of milk and dairy products in his diet. Certainly it would give the diagnosis greater credibility if it was known that Darwin had an unusually high lactose-containing diet. This proves to be the case. In a recently published collection of Emma Darwin's recipes, the authors state, 'Darwin loved sweet things. Emma's recipe book includes more than sixty puddings, not counting the jams and preserves… Emma uses *plenty of milk, lots of cream* [our italics] and eggs, and fruit'.[46] Indeed, the household seems to have used dairy products to excess. Emma wrote to her daughter Henrietta: 'Our strawberries are grand, and there are some in the house who certainly enjoy them. I found we were spending 5s. [shillings] a day on cream and milk, so Mrs B. and I were equally shocked and are not going to be so magnificent [sic]'.[47] Charles was equally shocked and embarrassed by the family's use of cream when he took his sickly son, William, to visit Robert Darwin, Charles' father, in Shrewsbury. Charles wrote back to Emma, 'I felt quite ashamed, at finding out, what I presume you did not know anymore than I did, that he has half a cup of cream every morning – which my Father (who seemed rather annoyed) says he believes is one of the most injurious things we could have given him'.[48]

We can conclude that Darwin's diet had a high sugar, high lactose content – when it was under the management of his wife. The latter point is an important one. Darwin's chronic illness began around the time he got married. Certainly, the main symptoms appear to have developed about a year after his marriage in January 1839. The first mention that he makes of 'periodical vomiting' is in June 1840, when he also complains of six months of 'very indifferent health'.[49] His health aboard the *Beagle*, when he must have had a lactose-poor diet over several years, was excellent apart from sea-sickness and a couple of episodes of fever in South America. Furthermore, a change in diet could explain how Darwin benefited from hydropathy. After his marriage, visits to hydropathic establishments were the only times that he spent a sustained period away from home. A tenet of all these hydropathic establishments was a 'healthy', and therefore restricted, diet. Darwin complained that Dr Gully 'allowed me a little milk to sop the stale toast in. At no time must I take any sugar, butter, spices tea bacon or anything good'.[50] The implication is that Gully normally did not allow him any milk. Darwin was particularly helped by a special diet prescribed by Dr Bence Jones. According to Darwin, the diet consisted of 'scanty amounts of toast and meat', but he was sure that it had done him good. He told Hooker, 'I have been half starved to death & am 15lb lighter, but I have gained in walking power & my vomiting is immensely reduced'.[51] Despite its obvious efficacy, the rigorous dietary regime was eventually put aside and Darwin returned to his 'comfort foods' – especially the puddings and the sweets.

A close relationship between Darwin's illness and diet is in keeping with his health record while in Ilkley. He arrived from home in poor health, and after thirteen days in the hydropathic establishment under Dr Smith's dietary regime, he felt better. He then moved out to join Emma, and at North House he would, to some extent, have slipped into the family's usual dietary habits, whereupon he developed skin rashes and other problems. After five weeks he moved back into the hotel, and over the last ten (lactose-restricted) days, he enjoyed walks on the moor and 'inhaling health'. His good health rapidly faded when he got back to Down House, as he returned to home cooking, and a high-lactose diet.

Although there are pitfalls in retrospective diagnosis,[52] we believe there is much to commend lactose intolerance as the cause of Darwin's illness. If this diagnosis is correct, we must conclude that Darwin lacked the genetic mutation that would have enabled him to tolerate lactose and to utilise it as a nutrient into adult life. Darwin's genetic make-up, and the consequent enigmatic illness, represents a failure to conform to an adaptation (persistent lactase production) that, through natural selection, prevails in the general population. Darwin, as with much else in his remarkable life, did not follow the herd.

Notes

1   C.D. to Charles Kingsley, 30 November 1859; Correspondence, 7, p. 407.

2   C.D. to Charles Lyell, 2 December 1859; Correspondence, 7, p. 409.

3   C.D. to John Lubbock, 14 December 1859; Correspondence, 7: p. 433. In a letter written on the same day to J.D. Hooker, he makes an almost identical comment, '…the last 10 days at Ilkley did me much good; though I have retrograded since being at home, from having had rather an extra heavy dose of things to do'. (C.D. to J.D. Hooker, 14 December 1859, Correspondence; 7: p. 432).

4   C.D. to Asa Gray, 21 December 1859; Correspondence, 7, p. 440.

5   C.D. to J.D. Hooker, 21 December 1859; Correspondence, 7, p. 441.

6   C.D. to Leonard Horner, 23 December 1859; Correspondence, 7, p. 444.

7   C.D. to W.D. Fox, 25 December 1859; Correspondence, 7, p. 449

8   C.D. to J.D. Dana, 30 December 1859, Correspondence; 7, p. 462.

9   The first hydropathic institute in the United States was opened in 1844 in New York by Dr Joel Shew, a physician who had undergone treatment by Priessnitz at Gräfenberg. In 1845, Shew became manager of a similar establishment in New Lebanon Springs, New York. He contributed to The Water-Cure Journal, and was the author of several works on water treatment. (see http://famousamericans.net/joelshew/). By 1860, there were over 200 residential hydropathic establishments in the United States. See S.E. Cayleff, 'The history of the hydropathic movement in the United States', in Encyclopedia of Complementary Health Practice, ed. by C.C. Clark, R.J. Gordon, B. Harris and C.O. Helvie, Springer Publishing, New York, 1999. pp. 105-107.

10   C.D. to Charles Lyell, 25 June 1860; Correspondence, 8, p. 265.

11   C.D. to W.D. Fox, 4 September 1863; Correspondence, 11, p. 620.

12   C.D. to J.D. Hooker, 4 October 1863; Correspondence, 11, p. 646.

13   Emma Darwin to W.E. Darwin, 28 October 1863; Correspondence, 11, p. 654.

14   Colp Jr., R., Darwin's Illness (University Press of Florida, Gainsville, Florida: 2008) p. 114.

15   The ICD-10 Classification of Mental and Behavioural Disorders, Clinical Descriptions and Diagnostic guidelines. World Health Organisation. http://www.who.int/classifications/icd/en/bluebook.pdf p. 129.

16   Kempf, E.J., Psychopathology (C.V. Mosby, St. Louis: 1920) p.209; Hubble, D., 'The evolution of Charles Darwin', Horizon, 1946; 14: p. 84 ; Good, R., 'The life of the shawl', Lancet, 1954; i: p.106; Graber, R.G., and Miles, L.P., 'In Defence of Darwin's Father'. History of Science, 1988; 26: p. 97-102; Bowlby, J., Charles Darwin: A New Life. (W.W. Norton & Co., New York: 1991) pp. 460-2; and others.

17   Pickering, G., *Creative Malady, The Invalid Recluse* (Oxford University Press, New York: 1974) pp. 53-70.

18   Medawar, P.B., *Darwin's Illness, The Art of the Soluble* (Methuen, London: 1967) p. 114.

19   Barloon, T.J. and Noyes, R., 'Charles Darwin and Panic Disorder', *Journal of the American Medical Association*, 1997; 277: pp. 138-41.

20   Lieb, J., 'The paradoxical advantages and disadvantages of natural selection: The case history of Charles Darwin'. *Medical Hypotheses*, 2007; 69: pp. 1375-77.

21   Adler, S., 'Darwin's illness', *Nature*, 1959; 184: 1102-3.

22   Kohn, L.A., 'Charles Darwin's chronic ill health', *Bulletin of the History of Medicine*, 1963; 37: 239-56; de Beer, G., *Charles Darwin: Evolution by Natural Selection* (Doubleday & Co. Garden City, New York: 1964) pp. 115-17; Medawar, P.B., 'Darwin's illness', *Annals of Internal Medicine*, 1964; 61: p. 782; Adler, S., 1959; 184: p. 1103.

23   Umezawa, E.S., et al., 'Chagas' disease'. *Lancet*, 2000; 357: pp. 797-99.

24   Darwin, C. *Journal of Researches into the Geology and Natural History of the Various Countries visited during the Voyage of H.M.S. Beagle round the World* (Everyman's Library, Dent, London: 1906) p. 316.

25   Woodruff, A.W., 'Darwin's health in relation to his voyage to South America'. *British Medical Journal*, 1965; 1: pp. 745-50.

26   The principal alternative diagnoses are arsenic poisoning (see Colp Jr., R., 2008; pp. 149-54); Myalgic encephalomyelitis – 'M.E.' (Field, E.J., 'Darwin's illness', *Lancet*, 1990; 336: p. 826); Multiple allergy syndrome (Smith, F., 'Charles Darwin's ill-health', *Journal of the History of Biology*, 1990; 23: pp. 443-59); Ménière's disease (Gordon, A.G., 'The duelling diagnoses of Darwin', *Journal of the American Medical Association*, 1997; 277: p. 1276); and Crohn's disease (Orrego, F., and Quintana, C., 'Darwin's illness: a final diagnosis', *Notes and Records of the Royal Society*, 2007; 61: pp. 23-9).

27   The first suggestion of lactose sensitivity as a cause was made by Campbell, A.K., and Matthews, S.B., 'Darwin's illness revealed', *Postgraduate Medical Journal*, 2005; 81: pp. 248-51.

28   Ingham, C.J.E., et al., 'Lactose digestion and the evolutionary genetics of lactase persistence', *Human Genetics*, 2007: pp. 311-13.

29   Lomer, M.C.E., Parkes, G.C., and Sanderson, J.D., 'Lactose intolerance in clinical practice – myths and realities', *Alimentary Pharmacology and Therapeutics*, 2008; 27: pp. 93-103.

30   Waud, J.P., Matthews, S.B., and Campbell, A.K., 'Measurement of breath hydrogen and methane, together with lactase phenotype, defines the current best practice for investigation of lactose sensitivity', *Annals of Clinical Biochemistry*, 2008; 45: 50-58.

31   Harrington, L.K., and Mayberry, J.F., 'A re-appraisal of lactose intolerance', *International Journal of Clinical Practice*, 2008; 62: pp. 1541-46.

32   Talley, N.J., and Spiller, R., 'Irritable bowel syndrome: a little understood organic bowel disease?' *Lancet*, 2002; 360: pp. 555-64.

33   Di Stefano, M., et al., 'Visceral hypersensitivity and intolerance symptoms in lactose malabsorption', *Neurogastroenterology and Motility*, 2007; 19: pp. 887-95.

34   Sheehan, W., Meller, W.H., and Thurber, S., 'More on Darwin's illness: Comment on the final diagnosis of Charles Darwin', *Notes and Records of The Royal Society*, 2008; 62: pp. 205-9.

35   C.D. to C.S. Wedgwood, May 1838; Correspondence, 2, p.85.

36   C.D. to J.D. Hooker, May 1845; Correspondence, 3, p. 186.

37   C.D. to J.D. Hooker, 20-22 February 1864; Correspondence, 12, p. 57.

38   'Notes on Darwin's Heath', Appendix IV, Correspondence, 13: p. 482.

39 Colp Jr., R., 2008. p. 175.

40 For example, Emma Darwin to W.D. Fox, 29 September 1863; Correspondence, 11, p. 643 n. 4.; and C.D. to John Chapman, 7 June 1865; Correspondence, 13, p. 179.

41 C.D. to W.D. Fox, 7 July 1849; Correspondence, 4, p. 224.

42 C.D. to W.D. Fox, 24 October 1852; Correspondence, 5, p. 100.

43 C.D. to H. Bence Jones, 3 January 1866; Correspondence, 14, p. 4.

44 H. Bence Jones to C.D., 10 February 1866; Correspondence, 14, p. 52.

45 Browne, J., *Charles Darwin: The Power of Place*, (Jonathan Cape, London: 2002) p. 264.

46 Bateson, D., and Janeway, W., *Mrs Darwin's Recipe Book*. (Glitterati Inc., New York: 2008) p. 115.

47 It seems likely that the word 'magnificent' is a transcription error and it should be 'munificent' – great generosity. 5 shillings was an enormous amount to spend each day on milk and cream. It would be equivalent to over £20 in today's values. From Litchfield, H. 1915. v. 2, p. 262.

48 C.D. to Emma Darwin, 1 July 1841; Correspondence, 2, p. 294.

49 C.D. to W.D. Fox, 7 June 1840; Correspondence, 2, p. 270.

50 C.D. to Susan Darwin, 19 March 1849; Correspondence, 4, p. 224.

51 C.D. to J.D. Hooker, 28 September 1865, Correspondence; 13; p. 246. See also footnote 4, p. 247, 'He had numerous bouts of sickness in August but only two in September' (on the Bence-Jones diet).

52 Cunningham, A. 'Identifying disease in the past: Cutting the Gordian knot'. *Asclepio*, 2002; 54: pp. 13-34.

Index

Other titles published by The History Press

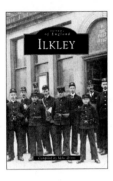

Ilkley: Images of England
MIKE DIXON

A 'rustic and inaccessible' village at the beginning of Queen Victoria's reign, Ilkley grew to become a fashionable inland spa and developed apace as both a health resort and an attractive residential town. Through this remarkable collection of over 200 images we see the town of Ilkley develop over the years. Full and descriptive captions accompany each picture making this a thoroughly enjoyable and informative read for everyone who knows the area.

978 0 7524 1507 9

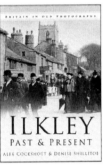

Ilkley Past & Present
ALEX COCKSHOTT & DENISE SHILLITOE

With the help of old photographs, this book traces the history of Ilkley from being a small town to a place of tourist attraction. Referred to in the 'Domesday Book', it was a small agricultural village for centuries; all this changed when the potential of the local waters was realised in the eighteenth century, and Ilkley became known as a spa.

978 0 7509 3922 5

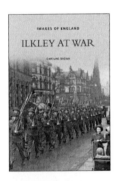

Ilkley at War: Images of England
CAROLINE BROWN

In the nineteenth century, Ilkley prospered as an inland spa resort. During the war years the grand hydros and hotels were adapted for war-time uses; hostels for evacuees and bases for government offices and the military. This book describes how Ilkley, Burley and Menston adapted to all the changing circumstances of a community at war.

978 0 7542 4191 7

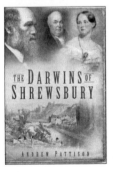

The Darwins of Shrewsbury
ANDREW PATTISON

Many people have written biographies of Charles Darwin, but the story of his family and roots in Shrewsbury is little known. This book, containing original research, fills that gap. The stories of Charles' five siblings are detailed, and there is a wealth of local material, such as information on Shrewsbury School and its illustrious headmaster, Samuel Butler. The book is fully illustrated with contemporary and modern pictures, and will be of interest to anyone wanting to discover more about the development of Shrewsbury's most famous son.

978 0 7524 4867 1

Visit our website and discover thousands of other History Press books.
www.thehistorypress.co.uk